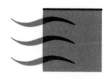
INTRODUCTION TO

HEALTH CARE DELIVERY AND RADIOLOGY ADMINISTRATION

Stephen S. Hiss, RT, MS

The Chester County Hospital
West Chester, PA

W.B. SAUNDERS COMPANY

A Division of Harcourt Brace & Company

Philadelphia London Toronto
Montreal Sydney Tokyo

W.B. SAUNDERS COMPANY

A Division of Harcourt Brace & Company

The Curtis Center
Independence Square West
Philadelphia, PA 19106

Library of Congress Cataloging-in-Publication Data

Hiss, Stephen S.
    Introduction to health care delivery and radiology administration /
Stephen S. Hiss
        p.   cm.
    ISBN 0-7216-5314-6
    1. Radiology, Medical—Management.   2. Medical care—United
States.   3. Insurance, Health—United States.   4. Hospitals—
Radiological services—Management.   I. Title.
    [DNLM: 1. Delivery of Health Care—United States.   2. Hospital
Administration—United States.   3. Insurance, Health—United States.
4. Quality Assurance, Health Care—United States.   5. Radiology—
organization & administration.   W 84 AA1 H65i 1997]
R898.H57   1997
362.1′77—dc20
DNLM/DLC   96–21134

INTRODUCTION TO HEALTH CARE DELIVERY
AND RADIOLOGY ADMINISTRATION   ISBN 0–7216–5314–6

Printed in the United States of America

Last digit is the print number: 9   8   7   6   5   4   3   2   1

To my two daughters
Kimberly, for her love of music,
and Laura, for her love of dance;
and to my wife Pat,
for her genuine belief in the human spirit.

PREFACE

They say we must improve health care delivery in the United States, and do it at a lower cost. Who says so? Certainly not everyone. Who is right and who is wrong? Some say the system is the best in the world, even the envy of the world. What parts need to be improved? Who will do it? What are the priorities and agendas of these engineers of change? Do the seers look beyond the statistics, and can they feel and care about the second and third order of impact their solutions will have on an unsuspecting population who can perhaps least afford this landslide of change, and who may have little ability to lobby on their own behalf?

Changing the health care delivery system goes well beyond debates in Washington. It represents and embodies a new set of personal standards and values with regard to our own people as services are balanced against cost. As a result, what we have come to recognize as anchor points and benchmarks for quality of service will be altered significantly in the future. Many have been served perhaps excessively at the health care table, whereas others may have died because of the system's flaws. A strong argument can be made that the excesses have been so great that their moderation will not significantly affect the *haves* as the *have nots* receive the new services they deserve. The principal questions may well be how intelligently this moderation can be engineered and defined and how effectively it can be administered.

None of these issues will be determined by one person or even a small group of people. The complex mosaic of expenses and services that are the bits and pieces of our current health delivery system will ultimately be redefined in the private sector on a more-or-less free-market basis, as subscribers (the patients) evaluate and vote their preference by signing on with one competing managed care organization or another. If the primary struggle lies in these people choosing their managed care organization on the basis of the coverage offered, other battles will be fiercely fought among providers as *they* maneuver to win contracts with the payers and managed care organizations of the future. The hospitals and their staffs that win these battles will be the facilities that have defined the most cost-effective services.

As health care administrators poise their respective facilities and set strategies for a successful campaign to win these managed care contracts, the individual health care worker has a much larger and more determining role to play than he or she ever had in the past. The focus of this text is to provide the reader with a comprehensive overview of the concepts driving health care delivery today. It also provides critical insight into how these changes are likely to affect the health care worker as we prepare ourselves for future demands. It has been said more than once that knowledge is power; today, knowledge has become a vital survival tool that can benefit individual careers as well as the organizations we work for. As providers face greater risks and possible demise by losing payer contracts, health care workers are at equal risk if they do not understand their industry and the significance of their individual efforts. The individual efforts of those who have direct contact with patients and those who administer and drive new strategies and changes will be *jointly,* not individually, responsible for the success of any given facility.

The inertia of the "more is better philosophy" of his huge industry will not be altered overnight. It will happen as intelligent strategies are engineered and carried out by those who see and understand the new ground rules well before the decree is issued, and the information in this text provides direction in that regard. Readers will benefit most if they approach the material and concepts presented with a willing and open mind, and with a clear understanding of their individual roles and new responsibilities as agents and advocates for positive change—rather than as protectors of the status quo.

Stephen S. Hiss, RT, MS

CONTENTS

THREE

The Hospital as an Organized and Integrated System 75

FOUR

Financial Aspects of Hospital Management 101

FIVE

The Health Care Insurance System 135

SIX
Quality of Care **155**

SEVEN
Introduction to Radiology
Department Management **179**

EIGHT
Logistics and Intradepartmental
Dependencies 203

NINE
Radiology Management **219**

TEN
Radiology Services Provided by Freestanding Facilities **261**

ONE

Historical Overview of Health Care Delivery in the United States

OBJECTIVES FOR STUDY

After reading this chapter, the student will

- ▶ Appreciate the origin, scope, and skill of medical care in the United States from the late 1700s to the early 1900s.

- ▶ Appreciate past conditions under which medical care was given and how the initial level of care evolved to current levels.

- ▶ Understand the various philosophies of caregivers that evolved in the late 1700s and through the 1800s.

- ▶ Appreciate how medical schools evolved into today's university-based, highly specialized, research-driven facilities.

- ▶ Appreciate how hospitals were founded during the 1800s.

- ▶ Understand the evolution of city, state, and federal government involvement in health care.

MEDICAL CARE FROM 1700 TO 1920

In Colonial America in the early 1700s, medical care was provided in an informal style. There were no established facilities, and caregivers were few. In fact, primary medical care was generally given in the home by people who had nothing more than a keen interest in taking care of others—and few if any available instructors to learn from (Fig. 1-1). Very few, perhaps fewer than 10, formally trained physicians were available to take care of the ill and injured along the entire eastern seaboard (Fig. 1-2). The colonists developed individual interests in learning about medical care, but the information available to them was scanty. Books on the subject often were not written by physicians at all, but by clerics and lay citizens who had developed an interest in writing about medical care delivery and who logged and wrote about their experiences (Fig. 1-3). Books such as *The Poor Planter's Physician,* by John Tennent, and *Primitive Physic,* written in 1764 by John Wesley, Founder of the Methodist societies and Methodism, provide some insights into the level of medical educational expertise available at this time.

By the mid-1700s, other, more formal documentation had become available, and a gradual awareness that people could make a more meaningful impact on their state of health, even in this primitive environment, began to unfold. In addition, the population continued to increase, and the number of trained physicians increased as well. With the arrival of these trained physicians from Europe, a more formalized approach began to develop (Fig. 1-4). Philosophical disagreements as to how much medical care should be depended on as opposed to "natural healing" were argued with increased intensity. Various members of the clergy began to question the role of physicians, particularly when initial questions of drug interventions of any kind were under consideration. Also, isolation hospitals appeared shortly after 1700, and were followed by inoculation hospitals by the mid-

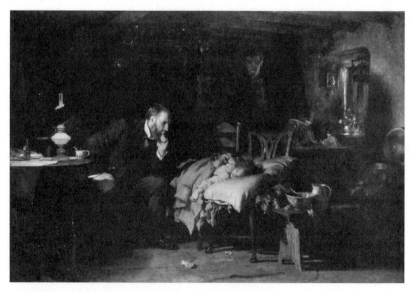

▶ **FIGURE 1–1** Early medical care was limited to basic treatment and took place in the home. (Source: National Library of Medicine.)

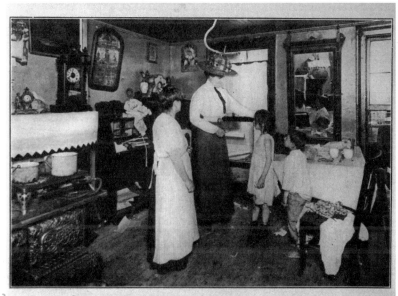

The school nurse is the most efficient link between the school and the home.

▶ **FIGURE 1-2** Often primary caregivers or "healers" were women who informally provided care and remedies based on their own experience, interest, compassion for the sick. (Source: National Library of Medicine.)

1700s. Williamsburg, Virginia founded one of the first institutions for the mentally ill in 1773.

Around 1730, a few trained physicians began to offer formal courses in the treatment of diseases and injuries in a few fledgling cities that had been established along the east coast from Boston to Philadelphia. These programs eventually led to a degree program called the Bachelor of Medicine. Many physicians took patients who needed continuous treatment at their own homes. Other, more advanced programs developed later that led to the degree of Medical Doctor (MD). By the time the Revolutionary War had begun, there were approximately 47 physicians in the eastern United States, 7 of whom had been awarded the MD degree. However, approximately 40 physicians were practicing with Bachelor of Medicine Degrees. With these medical degree programs in their infancy, the need to formalize medical training had become urgent, and efforts to develop more programs increased. By 1830 the country's first five medical schools had graduated a total of 250 doctors. The need for improved communications among these individuals also became obvious. An outbreak of yellow fever in Philadelphia in 1735 brought forth the first medical journal in Colonial America, *Medical Respiratory,* and a new medical society, the Medical Society of Boston, was founded in 1736. In 1766, the New Jersey Medical Society was formed in New Brunswick. These societies also began to encourage the establishment of facilities that could provide basic care outside the home. The first designated medical care facilities began to appear in Philadelphia, at Pennsylvania Hospital. It was established primarily to care for the mentally ill, and broadened its services to include general medicine. Pennsylvania

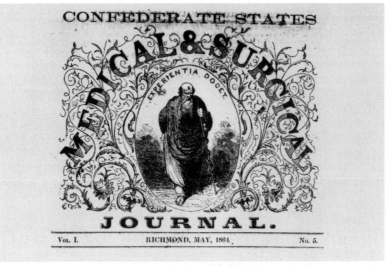

▶ **FIGURE 1-3** (A) An early medical journal. (B) Many advertisements in early medical journals were written by people about treatments they had developed and used. (Source for A and B: National Library of Medicine.)

Hospital remains today as the oldest and first formally established hospital in the United States. Dr. Thomas Bond (1712–1782), in collaboration with Benjamin Franklin, founded Pennsylvania Hospital in 1751. John Morgan founded the first medical college, the College of Philadelphia, in 1765. These, among other important contributions to medicine, gave Philadelphia recognition as the cradle of medicine in America.

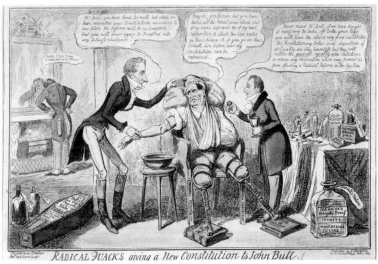

A

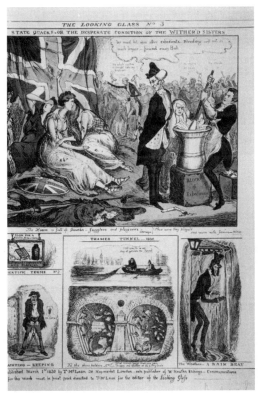

B

▶ **FIGURE 1–4** (A, B) Caricatures of quackery in medicine, which was common in the early years. (Source: National Library of Medicine.)

GRADUAL FORMATION AND FOCUS OF MEDICAL CARE

As the population began to increase more rapidly in the mid-1700s, the demand for medical care also increased. However, the demand was greater than the supply of facilities and fully trained caregivers. As a result, a difference in the quality of care provided among the wealthy and the poor, and the urban and the rural population, began to widen. Practically all the medical care of the period was provided as charity. Physicians took what their patients could give in money, favors, free labor, free goods, food, or animals. The most experienced and highly trained caregivers (MDs) were most accessible to those who could pay with cash, however, and to those who lived in or near a concentration of people, primarily in the developing cities. For the most part, those who did not fall into this paying urban group received medical care from "folk" practitioners.

As a continuing accommodation to the expanding population, additional health care facilities began to emerge. By 1770, approximately 100 designated health care facilities were scattered over the eastern seaboard (Fig. 1-5). Their initial and principal mission was to provide for the homeless and destitute. In addition, efforts toward providing the most basic health care were carried out. Almost all of these almshouses were essentially funded through meager appropriations from various provincial governments, but most funds came from private donations and foundations that were slowly emerging. The facilities were operated primarily by volunteers, including physicians who had full training while others had no training at all. On-the-job training for medical practitioners was the rule rather than the exception. Beyond providing basic medical care, these facilities also provided shelter for the homeless. As indicated earlier, Pennsylvania Hospital was an outgrowth of one of these facilities providing both medical care and shelter for the homeless in 1751 (Fig. 1-6). Oth-

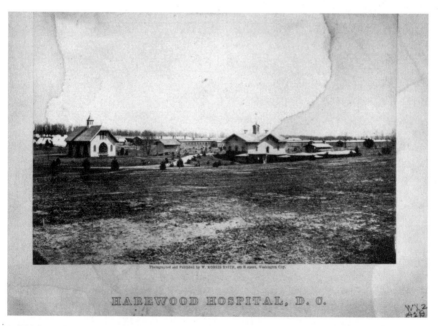

▶ **FIGURE 1–5** Early military health care facilities (1863) in many instances led the way in establishing a model for civilian facility-based health care. (Source: National Library of Medicine.)

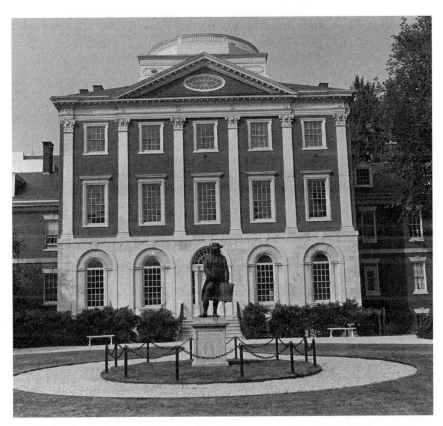

▶ **FIGURE 1-6** Original building of the Pennsylvania Hospital, Philadelphia, founded in 1751 by Benjamin Franklin. (Courtesy of Pennsylvania Hospital, The Ayer Clinical Laboratory.)

er major cities along the eastern seaboard built facilities having similar missions. However, by the late 1700s, several of the provincial governments among the colonies had accepted some responsibility for the payment of medical expenses for merchant seamen, through funds collected from shipmasters. This occurred because the colonies were so dependent on shipping for supplies from Europe that healthy sailors were considered vital to the success of the colonies.

Many hospitals were started by core groups of physicians who were able to appropriate funds from their own resources and from local citizens of financial means (Fig. 1-7). Foundations also helped in this regard. The community hospital in Chester County, Pennsylvania, is typical of many hospitals that were founded during the middle and late 1800s. Figure 1-8 shows the community's proclamation for a hospital to be located in the town of West Chester to serve residents of that community and surrounding area. Excerpts from various articles from the local newspaper of those times included articles that indicate the nature and scope of services provided at these community facilities. Moreover, on reading these articles, one can clearly detect the strong and intimate sense of ownership the community had in providing and receiving health care. One can also appreciate the sense of charity that was the seed of the nation's concept of entitlement, which became law through Medicare legislation in the mid-1960s. A careful reading and interpretation of these articles also pro-

For a Hospital

Report of Committee of the Chester Medical Society, Appointed to Prepare and Issue a Circular to the People of Chester County.

Report

In response to a resolution adopted at a public meeting held May 19th at Library Hall, in West Chester, requesting the Chester County Medical Society to prepare a circular for general distribution among the citizens of the county, setting forth the need of establishing a hospital in this place for the treatment of all medical and surgical cases that would be likely to be benefited by to benefited from such care, the undersigned beg leave to submit the following.

1. There is no such institution within the limits of the county, with the single exception of the almshouse, and, excellent as this institution is, its isolated position and meagre conveniences poorly fit it for the purpose of a general hospital. In addition to these objections we find great difficulty in inducing the sick to the almshouse and thus receive the brand of paupers.

2. We send many cases annually to the Philadelphia hospitals, where they are separated from their homes and friends. They often incur serious injury from the necessary changes incident to transportation, and the way in these cases may be very injurious.

3. West Chester is more accessible to most of Chester County than is Philadelphia and we think it is the way of West Chester County to care for her own sick and injured within her own limits. Over fifty cases were sent to Philadelphia hospitals during the past year.

4. There are now many cases of incurable disease which are a burden to the county and to charitable people which could have been restored to health and rendered self supporting in the early stages of their trouble, if it had been possible to place them under the conditions indispensable to their proper treatment.

5. A majority of the cases treated in this hospital, as in all hospitals of its class, wold be acute and chronic medical cases and chronic conditions requiring operative interference. Those suffering from recent incidents would form a small part of the total number. Any one familiar with the Philadelphia hospitals knows how difficult it is to obtain admission there for those suffering from chronic diseases.

6. It is not the poor alone that would be benefited by a general hospital. Many well-to-do people would make themselves of its advantages when they could not have proper care at home. Such would be a source of revenue for its support.

7. All classes would be benefited by the establishment in its connection of a training school for nurses. The time has come for the appreciation of trained and skilled labor and nowhere are its results more striking than in the sick room.

It has been proposed that the contribution of one hundred dollars constitute a life membership and entitle the contributor to one vote annually in the management. One hundred dollars annually entitles the contributor to one bed in the hospital.

Four thousand dollars ($4,000) shall constitute the endowment of a perpetual bed.

Five dollars ($5) annually shall entitle the contributor to one vote in the management.

Additional contributions on the same basis.

The co-operation of the citizens of the whole county is desired, as it is intended that the benefits of this hospital shall be as freely extended to the residents of the remote parts of the county as to those in the vicinity of West Chester.

▶ **FIGURE 1–7** Proclamation and founding of the new Chester County Hospital. (Source: Archives of The Chester County Historical Society.)

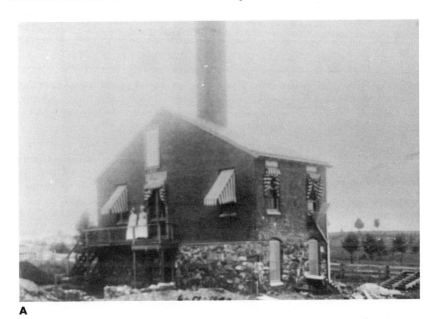

A

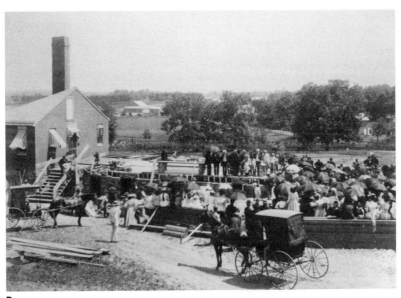

B

▶ **FIGURE 1-8** (A) The original building of a community hospital in West Chester, Pennsylvania: The Chester County Hospital. (B) Construction phase of the hospital at West Chester, Pennsylvania. (Source for A and B: National Library of Medicine.)

vides a window toward understanding the lack of a strong "business" motive for running these early hospitals. Within the first year of its existence, the "pride" of the community was in financial trouble because the demand for services had already moved beyond the capability of the facility; the facility was a dependent of the State Board of Charities, and private donations were increased. A generation of "good" health care managers championed these charity responsibilities and in doing so had to find and learn to live with alternative revenue sources. Even as managed care evolves today, the fundamental imbalance of supply, demand, and resources has not changed. This created a mind-set among the boards of managers and facility supervisors of the day that deficit spending was a necessity in providing health care. Health care managers through the years felt somewhat insulated from taking the initiative to adopt aggressively many fundamental "business" practices. In fact, administrators have been strongly criticized for being reactionary, unconcerned with advocating a business attitude in their operations, too political, possessing tunnel vision, and so forth. This was in sharp contrast to tough-minded business non-health care entrepreneurs who had the luxury of being able to select their "customers" simply by choosing not to do business or to provide service without assurance of payment—moreover, payment at the asking price. This voluntary process of selection virtually guaranteed success to almost all non-health care providers, in contrast to the "charitable mission" of health care providers.

The following articles from a local paper were graciously provided by The Chester County Historical Society.

December 31, 1892
$15,000 To Be Asked For

The State Board of Charities has approved a bill which will come before the Legislature making for an appropriation of $15,000 for West Chester's new hospital. The bill asks for the appropriation for "the erection and maintenance of the said hospital for two years."

Dr. Bush and others of the committee had the amount asked raised from $10,000 to $15,000 by strenuous efforts with Mr. Biddle and others of the State Board of Public Charities. The bill has already been drafted and will be presented to the Legislature at an early day.

September 19, 1893
The Chester County Hospital

The physician's report for July, 1893
Patients in hospital July 5
Admitted during month 8
Discharged during the month 7
Operations performed. 4

Mary E. Cheyney
Chas. E. Woodward

June 5, 1894

. . . The average expense for maintaining the Hospital during the past year has been about $250 a month. For half of that time, however, the small building only was occupied. In our present enlarged quarters the capacity for patients being more than . . . the expenses will be proportionately increased.

The funds in hand were found to be inadequate for the expenses (the interest only from endowment funds being available), and it was thought advisable to borrow the sum of $5,000. . . . We have a well appointed building, a staff of efficient physicians ready to give their best efforts and experience to the work. We have a competent Matron, a corps of intelligent and promising nurses, all anxious to do their part. The wards are full of suffering men and women gratefully receiving the benefits of this institution; while others are waiting to come in. . . .

April, 1895
Monthly Meeting of the Board of Managers of the Chester County Hospital
. . . The report of the financial committee showed that the expenses are between $400 and $500 a month. . . .

November 9, 1900
The three members of the Board of Managers of the Chester County Hospital are in Philadelphia t-day, having gone there to present a petition to the State Board of Charities, which is in session in that city. They are Captain R.R. Cornwell, President of the Board, William Sharpless, Treasurer, and J. Preston Thomas, Secretary.

The needs of the institution will be told, and charts of the building, with statistics regarding the number of patients treated, and the expense of conducting business. The Board of Charities will hear this presentation, and will recommend a sum of money for the Legislature to appropriate if it sees fit.

After the first of the year the report will be made to the Legislature, and the members thereof from this county, Messers. Snyder, Coryell, Lack, Cope, and Fox, will be looked to for active work in behalf of a neat appropriation.

March 28, 1900
. . . two checks for $10 each in aid at the fund looking to the erection of a contagious ward at the Chester County Hospital. One comes from Mrs. Henry J. Biddle . . . , and the other from her daughter Miss Christine W. Biddle. In behalf of the projectors of the ward we give thanks for these subscriptions. The help is timely and now who will imitate the example? . . .

December 5, 1990
At yesterday's monthly meeting of the Board of Managers of the Chester County Hospital, a new form of admission card was adopted. It was also agreed that no patients will be accepted until certain rules have been complied with. This does not refer to emergency cases, which are admitted at any and all times. . . .

1. That the number of free patients in the wards at any one time excepting emergency cases, shall not exceed twenty. 2. That no patient except emergency cases, shall be admitted without having filled up and signed the admission blank which contains the rules and rates of admission. 3. That no patients shall be admitted free without having signed a statement that they are without means to pay for hospital care.

All the physicians of the county have been asked to co-operate in the enforcement of these rules and have been furnished with blank application cards or certificates of admission, which read as follows: . . . The object of asking patients what they can afford to pay is that they may feel the necessity of paying something even though it should be a small amount. It has frequently occurred that persons who were able to pay did not, and that patients who were receiving sick benefits from beneficial orders were enjoying good treatment at the hospital and using their sick benefits for other purposes.

THE MILITARY'S INFLUENCE ON THE ADVANCEMENT OF HEALTH CARE

The military had a significant influence on the evolution of the medical care system during this period. By 1818, the United States Army had developed a Central Department of Medicine. Military conflict contributed to the development of medical research in the dubious sense that war casualties forced health care professionals to develop and deliver new techniques for the care of a wide range of diseases and disabilities. This large infusion of patients provided significant impetus to advance medical science, and medical facilities and treatment techniques were made available on a much larger scale than would have otherwise occurred. The number of casualties from military conflict also created a demand for

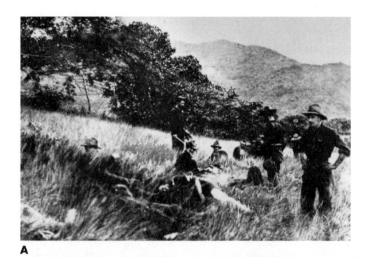

A

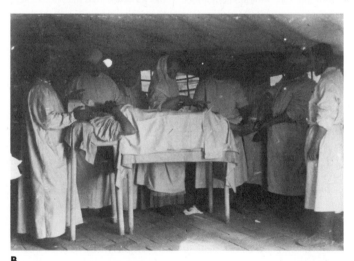

B

▶ **FIGURE 1–9** (A) A military field hospital around 1898. (B) Surgery at a field hospital around 1904. (Source for A and B: National Library of Medicine.)

more physicians and physicians' assistants, many of whom graduated into nursing positions (Fig. 1-9). In addition to war-related injuries, soldiers were subject to a variety of infectious diseases that sometimes spread quickly to the civilian population. New interest in identifying and testing for communicable diseases added additional pressure to expand services and education in health care delivery. It also succeeded in bringing government into the health care arena.

THE CHANGING ENVIRONMENT

By the mid-1800s, the U.S. economy began to move quickly to an urban manufacturing base, and new kinds of medical problems became evident as a large number of factory workers labored in close and unsanitary conditions (Fig. 1-10). In addition, new manufacturing processes used untested and uncontrolled toxic chemicals that caused a new order of illness, disease, and disabling injuries among workers in a greater variety than had been seen to date. In some instances, the large number of employee absences affected the productivity of the companies, and some factory owners resorted to hiring physicians to take care of their sick employees so they could return to work more quickly. As this practice increased, the level and nature of medical care provided by these factory owners received greater attention from local governments because of the growing number of people who were affected by these services. This appears to be the seed that many years later evolved into our present system of employer-funded benefit plans.

DIVERSITY IN TREATMENT PHILOSOPHIES

In the mid- and late 1800s, two very different philosophies of providing medical care began to emerge. One was known as the mainline group, characterized by a belief in dramat-

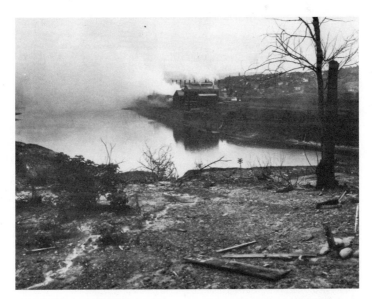

▶ **FIGURE 1-10** Clouds of smoke from factories often carried new toxins not only to workers, but also to the surrounding environment, which affected those who lived in the area. (Source: National Library of Medicine.)

ic treatments, including the practices of bloodletting and purging, that in some ways was mixed with spiritual beliefs. The "regulars" used more conventional methods to treat disease, including medication and techniques that were brought to the colonies by European physicians. The rivalry between these two groups became significant, but, eventually, the repulsive and morbid practices of the mainline group lost favor with the public, not to mention the questionable outcome of their services.

As the country's industrial movement developed further, more people had money to spend on medical care, and more and more physicians responded to the ever-increasing demand for the diagnosis and treatment of diseases. The disparity between the care given, however, to the "haves" and the "have nots" (those who had means to pay for medical services and those who did not) continued. This gap was generally overlooked by local governments and the fledgling federal government. Factory owners began to focus on the working population by establishing meager health care benefits as a means to reduce health related absenteeism. This manifested in a general awareness that treating diseases of workers had a higher priority than treating those of nonworkers. Government involvement accelerated as rapid concentrations of people in cities gave rise to significant outbreaks of infectious diseases such as cholera (Fig. 1-11). The Philadelphia Board of Health was one of the first established to monitor the number and severity of various diseases and mass outbreaks of illness. Before the Civil War, most states had the financial means but generally did not support medical care, except for specific conditions such as mental illness, pulmonary diseases, and confinement of people with highly contagious diseases.

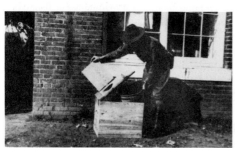

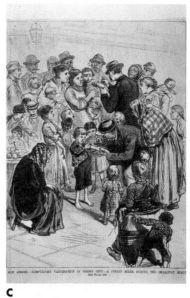

A

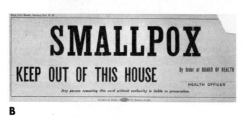

B   **C**

▶ **FIGURE 1–11** (A) A public health service worker places a container underneath an outside toilet, which was used in some instances before closed sanitation accommodations were required. (B) Public health service poster designating a quarantine area. Sometimes these posters were the primary method of treating and controlling contagious diseases. (C) Compulsory vaccination in the late 1800s. (Source for A–C: National Library of Medicine.)

Throughout the 1800s, there was a great deal of disagreement among government officials, factory owners, and the general population about how deeply government should be involved in medical care. The primary issues debated were (1) the degree to which public funding should be made available, (2) whether occurrence of disease, deaths, and other epidemiologic and demographic data should be recorded and whether this should be regulated through government programs, and (3) the extent to which legislation and funding should be infused into the system to force these activities, and, of course, (4) where the funds would come from. Ironically, these concerns have a very familiar ring today. Also in question was the growing issue of how future costs would be covered and whose responsibility they should be. By the late 1800s, most states had in place some mechanism for the registry of deaths, births, and an assortment of related statistics on infections and other common diseases. The signals were clear, however, that a more formalized health care provider program was needed. The overall health care problem had become too complex and too large to be ignored and handled in an adhoc manner.

THE ADVANCEMENT OF MEDICAL TRAINING AND EARLY SPECIALIZATION

The American Medical Association (AMA) was founded in 1847 to help develop the educational effort that was needed to support the growing demand for formally trained physicians. Several local medical societies also continued their missions to advance medical care by developing standards of practice and codes of ethics. Most of these were modeled after that advocated by Thomas Percival. By the late 1800s, several states had implemented licensure requirements for practicing physicians.

The need for medical training programs increased dramatically as the population became ever more concentrated in the cities. Between the mid-1700s and the early 1800s, five designated medical facilities had been founded to provide formalized training, which lead to a Medical Doctor degree (Fig. 1-12). Although the number of doctors available in the early 1800s was extremely small, the number of MDs who were practicing medicine by the middle and late 1800s grew to approximately 6,800. The physician's assistant also became increasingly important. A school of nursing was founded as a collaboration between the Nurse Society of Philadelphia and Dr. Joseph Warrington.

By the late 1800s, a concentration of specific diseases, ailments, and conditions demanded special attention and new study. This need was answered by a slowly emerging group of physicians whose principal interests lay in caring for patients with these particular conditions. As their efforts continued, the evolution of specialized medical practices was initiated, and by the turn of the century, specialists in surgery, lung, and mental illness were established. These were added to the already specialized fields of pharmacology and dentistry.

A SHIFT FROM REACTIVE TO PROACTIVE MEDICINE

Concepts of infection control and personal hygiene and an interest in preventive measures for controlling diseases began to emerge in the mid-1800s. Efforts in this regard, however, were usually limited to educating the population about hand washing and improving basic sanitary conditions. Previously, there was little understanding about such things as food processing, sanitation, rodents, and insects and their association with even the common diseases (Fig. 1-13).

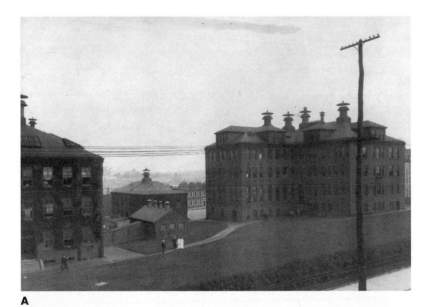

A

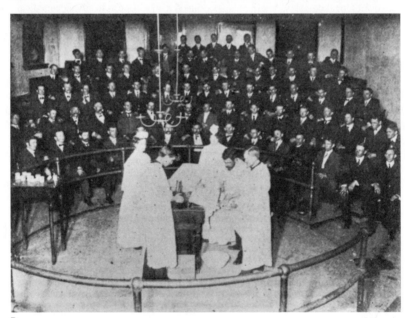

B

▶ **FIGURE 1–12** (A) One of the original medical science buildings at the Johns Hopkins campus, Baltimore, Maryland. (Courtesy of Johns Hopkins University, The Alan Mason Chesney Medical Archives.) (B) Typical surgical amphitheater of the early and mid-1800s. (Source: National Library of Medicine.)

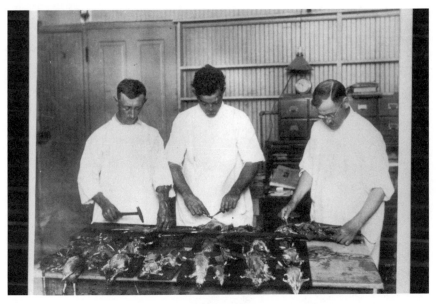

▶ **FIGURE 1–13** Public health workers inspecting rats for bubonic plague around 1914. (Source: National Library of Medicine.)

MORE THAN REGULAR MEDICINE

The trend toward more diverse treatment efforts continued, and these were practiced by a new order of medical sects. Their departure from "regular" medicine and conventional treatments with such modalities as "hydrotherapy" to flush the body of illness had gained some interest (Fig. 1-14). The Christian Science philosophy, another departure from "regular" medicine, advocated reliance on divine intervention and natural healing. Osteopathic care, advocated by Andrew Still, was a belief that certain illnesses and pain could be treated by manipulation of the body to relieve undue strain on the nervous system. Chiropractic treatment, introduced by Daniel Palmer in the late 1800s, derived from osteopathic principles. By the 1920s, 79 chiropractic schools had been established in the United States. Homeopaths, or "regulars," remained as the more conventional and largest group of physicians, however. They relied on techniques that led to a more scientific process for diagnosing illness, and on medications to the extent that they were available.

EARLY FORMS OF HOSPITAL CARE

By the last quarter of the 1800s, larger hospitals began to form. They were primarily funded through the encouragement of influential physicians, private philanthropists, and government officials. Medical societies also had a significant influence on this development. However, the concept of health care insurance certainly was not a topic of general discussion, and usually, such insurance was not available, much less affordable, to much of the population. Hospital bills at that time were paid by the patient or by companies that offered such assistance. In some instances, employers made loans to employees to pay for their health care services. By 1900, outpatient clinics began to form, in part subsidized by

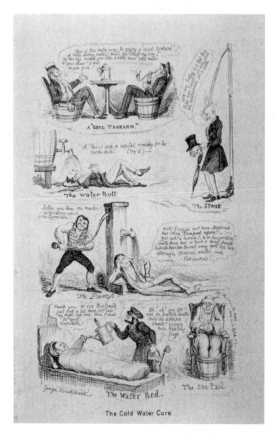

▶ **FIGURE 1-14** Six scenes depicting methods for administering the cold water cure used to "flush" disease from the patient (1782–1878). (Source: National Library of Medicine.)

local governments to help serve the needs of the poor. One of the most prominent of these early clinics was the Mayo Clinic in Rochester, Minnesota, established in 1889. It originated as a surgical facility but later expanded to provide general hospital services (Fig. 1-15). The Cleveland Clinic is another outstanding example.

Around the turn of the century, provision of medical care was emerging as a significant industry, with those directly involved as health care providers numbering in the hundreds of thousands. Formal training for all types of medical care practitioners and assistants was becoming a necessity as the amount of information involved in the diagnosis and treatment of illness started to explode, and as the time physicians had available to see each patient diminished. Universities accumulated large numbers of books and journals on medical care and began to structure new departments of medicine. Universities with new medical departments began to develop and merge medical facilities to attract promising individuals who wanted to teach in the medical departments. More research laboratories were formed, and fully developed medical schools with research centers began to emerge, during the early 1800s.

Because of the increasing need for ongoing medical care for soldiers, the United States Army had built a highly regarded medical library that was among the world's largest. The widespread desire to learn more about medicine had generated vast numbers of printed materials by the turn of the century, and the formation of medical research departments within universities spawned other specialties, such as physiology, biology, and a new and ac-

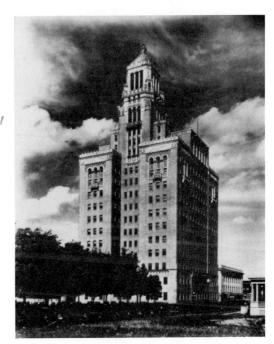

► **FIGURE 1-15** An early photo of the main building at the Mayo Clinic, Rochester, Minnesota. (Source: National Library of Medicine.)

celerated form of pharmacology. The Walter Reed Medical School was a prominent military medical school facility in Washington D.C., and it later became recognized for its work toward the cure for typhoid fever.

ADMISSION PRACTICES AND OPERATIONAL STANDARDS OF EARLY MEDICAL SCHOOLS

Schools of medicine had been structured as free-standing operations. Harvard University, however, was the first to merge its medical school with the university in 1870 and was one of the first universities to establish standardized admission requirements. It was at about this time that a new emphasis in medicine led to significant concerns about the quality of training programs in medical education and research. The number and diversity of medical school programs had increased and the need for standardizing and credentialing these programs drew much attention. The Carnegie Foundation for the Advancement of Teaching commissioned studies at more than 100 universities and medical schools around the country to determine what level of operational standards and practices had been applied, not only to admissions, but also to ongoing teaching and research programs. The basic elements evaluated in this study were entrance requirements, size and skill levels of facility, financial status, laboratory facilities, and clinical resources. The findings of the Flexner Report, as it was called, deeply concerned the medical community, as well as the federal government, and resulted in a much sharper focus and concentration of interest among medical societies and a group of state and federal efforts to improve standards within university programs. As a result of this report, the entire medical education process went through significant changes that became the basis for today's medical education curriculum.

In 1889, the Johns Hopkins Hospital was founded. Johns Hopkins's history is replete with unique and creative initiatives for advancing medical education. It distinguished itself by how it organized its services, which became the model that many modern training programs would follow. It was the first hospital in the country to organize its medical services by discipline, to each of which a head or chief of service was appointed. The medical school opened in 1893. It was viewed as one of the most demanding medical education institutions with regard to selection criteria, as noted in a brief excerpt from the publication, *A Model of Its Kind:*

> *The opening of the medical school in October 1893 was announced at the university's Commemoration Day exercises the preceding February. Word spread beyond Hopkins in the intervening eight months. . . . On October 2, these sixteen brought their credentials to the university's Biological Laboratory for Welch's perusal. Welch must have been relieved to see so many applicants, for the Hopkins faculty had no idea how many students would be interested in enrolling in the new institution, and they were afraid that their stringent admission requirements would discourage or exclude prospective students. All sixteen applicants were admitted, three of whom were women.*

The AMA took more aggressive action in directing public policy to improve general medical school standards, accomplishing this by using its growing membership and strengthening political base to encourage government policies requiring medical schools to work toward more aggressive standards. In addition, individual efforts by prominent physicians to further this cause were made through personal acquaintance and influence with public officials at the local, state, and federal levels. Despite these contacts, relatively few significant, sweeping laws were passed regarding health care services compared with those seen between 1940 and the present. The legislation that was passed was more concerned with standardization of services, the development of medical ethics, and the criteria for collecting statistics.

RAPID INDUSTRIALIZATION, GROWING URBAN AREAS, AND DISEASE CONTROL

With the list of newly identified and treatable diseases growing at an accelerated rate, the need for a more structured delivery system to make these advances available to the public was apparent. By this time, a few large hospitals were firmly in place and had developed funding sources that included meager offerings from the government and, to a larger degree, donations from foundations, philanthropists, and alumni. Funding from companies in payment for services to their employees also increased, as did the number of patients who could pay out of pocket.

The numerous contagious diseases that had spread through the growing cities affected large numbers of people. In addition, there was continued public concern with pressure exerted by physicians for government at all levels to develop more effective human services and policies for infection control and improved sanitary conditions. Medical societies began to promote a significant philosophical change. For the first time, they began to emphasize prevention of certain diseases rather than just treatment. Physicians had viewed themselves as primarily "healers" rather than as preventers of disease. In part, this was probably because so little was known about the prevention of disease, and the concept of cause and effect in disease processes was rudimentary. The rate of new diseases, maladies, and epidemics that had swept through cities and into the countryside in the 1700s and 1800s created a significant drain on medical resources. In rural areas, disease for the most part continued to be addressed in a second-hand fashion compared with services that were available in the urban areas.

THE CHANGING ROLE OF WOMEN IN HEALTH CARE

With the growing emphasis on meeting the demands of an ever-growing and more diversified population, the bulwark of male domination in the medical community eventually began to give way and to recognize women. Women began to make significant inroads into providing primary care in the role of nursing and in several ancillary medical services. The age of technology had not yet come, and jobs other than nurses and physicians that required specific technical expertise were few. Women began to form their own medical societies and lobbied for admission to medical schools. The AMA tried to block them but finally acquiesced. In 1915, approximately 6% of those graduating from medical school were women.

THE ROLE OF GOVERNMENT AND MEDICAL SOCIETIES IN DEFINING HEALTH CARE POLICY

As outbreaks of deadly and debilitating communicable diseases occurred with increasing frequency and with grave consequence, public pressure forced the federal government to become more involved in the delivery of health care. The need for a more centrally controlled, or at least coordinated, effort for providing medical care to large numbers of people had become urgent by the late 1800s. Strong concern continued in some quarters, however, regarding the degree to which government should become involved in subsidizing and providing health care, particularly with regard to the appropriateness of setting public policy for health care. In short, government involvement in health care seemed to be an entirely inappropriate extension of government power. Government agencies, despite this sentiment, continued to grow and expand their influence, especially in the arena of providing services to the poor.

City governments were the first to respond by implementing social policy reforms for controlling communicable diseases, sanitation, and food preparation and storage. City health officers gradually demanded and received more information from physicians regarding the type and frequency of diseases they had been seeing. New restrictions on the preparation of foods were implemented, and guidelines were written requiring better methods for storing meats, poultry, and milk products. Many new health education programs were developed as well, aimed at primary caregivers, medical facilities, and the general population. The concept of food contaminated with germs and the association of germs with disease was not widely known to much of the population until the early 1900s. Most people had to be taught the importance of simple hand washing.

A greater emphasis on disease prevention began to take hold as increasing numbers of medical articles were published by newspapers, magazines, and medical journals addressing the dangers of improper food preparation and storage and the benefits of proper sanitation (Fig. 1-16). City governments continued to emphasize prevention of infectious diseases through precautions ranging from simple hand washing to improving waste management systems. Massachusetts formed one of the first state board of health agencies in 1869. This movement was spearheaded in the most heavily populated cities of the northeastern seaboard.

The federal government got more intensely involved in providing large-scale medical

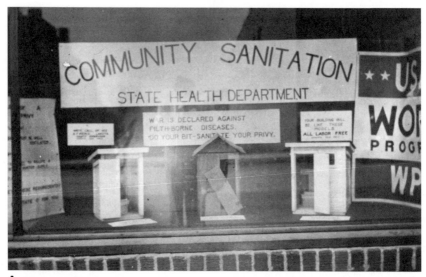

A

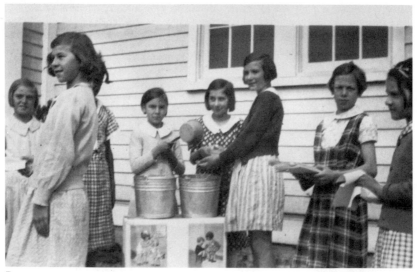

B

▶ **FIGURE 1-16** (A) Government display showing three model privies as a teaching aide for the general population to improve public and private sanitation practices. (B) Public health program to teach children the value of hand washing in controlling diseases. (Source for A and B: National Library of Medicine.)

services by forming the Marine Hospital Service in the early 1920s (Fig. 1-17). This medical service was designed to care for the seamen and longshoremen who carried goods from other countries into the United States. The Marine Hospital Service later expanded to include medical care for Native Americans, federal prisoners, and minors. Eventually, this effort became the Central Health Care Agency for the United States and was given a cabinet position. It was later renamed the Public Health Service. Its mission was redefined to include a broader scope of responsibilities, including (1) advancement of nutrition through health care, (2) monitoring activities of companies that offered health care insurance, and (3) monitoring activities of philanthropic foundations that supported medical matters. Through this cabinet position, the federal government also commissioned medical research studies at established universities, including Johns Hopkins and Harvard.

Some of the large insurance companies began to support health care facilities by providing medical information and analysis of the data they collected about their subscribers' illnesses. Several major philanthropic foundations, such as the Milbank Memorial Fund, con-

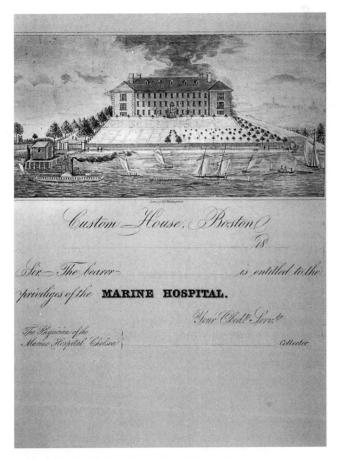

▶ **FIGURE 1-17** The Marine Hospital with ships in the foreground. (Source: National Library of Medicine.)

tributed significant amounts of money to key universities for the advancement of medical education and treatment of disease.

World War I provided an additional impetus to health care advancement. The treatment of highly infectious and contagious diseases such as cholera, yellow fever, and malaria was the military's primary concern. Provision of medical services to amputees and disabled veterans increased the government's involvement in health care, leading to increased utilization of military hospitals and the formation of the Veterans Hospital System. These facilities were designed to treat members of the armed services at no cost and were funded by the federal government through tax revenues. In World War II, more than 1 million soldiers were killed or injured, and approximately 700,000 soldiers sustained injuries that were eligible for care through these institutions. The demand for medical knowledge had accelerated once again.

AN AGING POPULATION AFFECTS THE DEMAND FOR HEALTH CARE SERVICES

By the mid-1940s, many of the highly contagious diseases that had threatened so much of the population were brought under control or eliminated. Medical treatment began to take on new types of challenges and illnesses as the average age of the population increased. Diseases such as cancer, heart disease, and vascular ailments, such as stroke, began to increase in incidence. With the study of more sophisticated diseases, a new set of medical requirements for diagnostic capabilities as well as treatment had to be developed. With the nuclear age came the technology of radioactive isotopes, which provided a new and exciting diagnostic tool, and diagnostic hardware based on radioisotopes was suddenly in great demand. Other, higher-energy, nuclear-age tools began to find applications in the treatment of cancers.

The same economic and demographic forces that had produced an older population also led to expanding tourism and immigration, which introduced diseases from other countries to the United States, such as the Hong Kong and Asian flus. These required new research for effective treatment and control. Advances in medical care continued to gain public attention as new cures and diagnostic tests became available that would have been unimaginable before the 1930s.

TOO MUCH GOVERNMENT, TOO LITTLE GOVERNMENT

The need to provide equal medical attention to people living in rural areas increased. It was also becoming clear to business owners that their costs would rise as their employees lobbied strenuously for more medical benefits. Competition to develop monitoring and controlling policies for medical services became intense, and large universities and the well-established medical societies were counseled to define public policy for medical care.

As the demand for specialists grew, so did their political strength. Fears among major medical societies such as the AMA (which advocated a rather generic point of view) of losing political control to newly formed societies of specialists increased. Such a loss of control to a growing number of specialists would certainly affect the AMA's political power and possibly its financial base, and friction among physicians began to grow. Surgeons, urologists, radiologists, cardiologists, and so forth, along with the American Nursing Association, attempted to advance the sentiments of their respective specialties at the expense of those of local societies or even the AMA. In all of this, the government's perceived role in extending health care to the disadvantaged became more confusing.

The rural population was characterized by low-paying or "no-pay" patients who still were not able to receive the benefits of highly skilled practices. In addition, the support services needed to diagnose and treat patients in these areas were not immediately available in numbers comparable to those in the city. Many of the smaller towns that did have modest but sufficient populations to support a small hospital or medical facility and staff had difficulty generating sufficient start-up funds to build.

GOVERNMENT TAKES A BIGGER BITE

In 1946, the United States initiated its first sweeping health care provider plan in the form of the Hill-Burton Act. With this law, the federal government contracted to provide funds in the form of grants and low-cost loans to build new hospitals or expand existing facilities in rural and urban areas where medical care was not sufficient. This act appropriated $3 million initially to serve hospital needs, and another $75 million for construction of new and expanded facilities over a five-year period. This greatly accelerated the expansion of the health care industry. In 1945, $85 million was spent on construction, which fueled a total of $353 million through 1953.

To get these funds, facilities had to meet specific criteria. The facilities that qualified to receive these funds were the beneficiaries of the country's first major federal government venture in establishing a delivery system within the framework of a focused health care provider plan. Its primary purpose was to make care available to the financially disadvantaged. Those individuals who fell into this category (as it was defined in the Act) could receive hospital care as needed without charge or at a declining scale of out-of-pocket expenses. These services included diagnostic procedures, hospitalization, and long-term medical care.

The Hill-Burton Act, with all its qualifiers, defined how much each hospital received based on the percentage of free care provided. Almost every hospital in the country scurried to find ways to gain access to these funds. Hospital administrators attempted to structure programs that would qualify their institutions for the most funding possible, while in some instances making the smallest commitment possible to taking nonpaying patients. The down side of receiving this funding was that hospitals had to open their financial books to an unprecedented extent, thus giving the federal government a much clearer view of how these institutions were charging for services, defining and managing operating costs, and managing their money in general. Some hospitals began to feel that they might have sold their souls and independence. From that point on, the government's influence (if not control) on hospitals would only become stronger as more government money became available in an industry whose means of generating income was much less than its means for controlling demand. As a result, hospitals were subjected to ever-increasing external control of their internal fiscal decisions. As time went on, it became unclear as to which of the two, hospitals or the government, was being manipulated the most. Loopholes and cracks in the legislative armor were found as hospitals tried to regain some of their lost control and independence, and revised government legislation attempted to close these loopholes as effectively as possible.

GROWTH OF COMMUNITY HOSPITALS

Even as this new window into the operations of hospitals opened, demand for better services increased. Hospitals grew rapidly in size and in number. Between 1946 and 1950, the number of beds increased by 356,000. Smaller community hospitals that were eligible for

Hill-Burton funding also grew as commercial insurance companies, such as Metropolitan and Prudential, provided more affordable coverage for those who could pay for premiums out of pocket. In addition, factories were contributing increased funding to health care group plans through employee benefit programs. The availability of this money in part separated those institutions whose administration established new programs and emerged as today's more prominent institutions.

LOCAL GOVERNMENT PROVIDES INITIAL INVOLVEMENT IN HEALTH CARE

The combination of a steadily increasing population and the demand for newly developing technology and medical services created tremendous friction between the providers and payers. The providers had been working with a fragmented and uncertain revenue stream, and payers saw their health care costs skyrocketing. It was clear to hospital administrators that strong financial management techniques had to be developed and implemented in an industry that had hitherto prided itself on philanthropy. Still, the disparity in medical services between paying and nonpaying patients continued. As a result, many municipalities, cities, and states began to form what turned out to be charity hospitals. These were fully owned and operated by city or state. The number of people with common ailments seeking medical care grew substantially, and by 1960, the number of so-called specialty hospitals also increased dramatically. These facilities provided specialized treatment for a single type of disease, such as heart and lung disease, cancer, or mental illness. Still others specialized in pediatric and women's health needs.

In the early 1950s, the development of high-tech diagnostic techniques accelerated at an even faster rate, with an emphasis on increased diagnostic medical care. As more technology came on line, more sophisticated diagnostic and treatment techniques were developed, resulting in an explosion of information. This in turn led to a dramatic increase in physician specialization and a decrease in "personalized" patient services. The introduction of catheters, wires, hoses, pumps, and other paraphernalia, which were developed to help patients, ironically also succeeded in pushing patients' personal needs into the background. The fervor surrounding new technology in the 1950s and 1960s merged with the excitement of the nuclear age of diagnostic testing in the early 1960s to ignite one of the most explosive periods of growth in medical science and diagnostic and treatment techniques the world had seen. The following list of total money spent annually for medical research gives an idea of the tremendous rate of growth. (See also Fig. 2-13.)

1950	$173 million
1955	$271 million
1960	$1,259 million
1965	$2,893 million
1975	$4,628 million

It was the beginning of the golden age of research and the development of new technologies and treatments. Private and government funding to support these efforts increased. Funding increased as universities merged and took financial control of their medical schools. By this time, many community hospitals that had been content to provide basic acute care began to see operational and financial advantages in affiliating with large medical schools. Other large community as well as tertiary care hospitals quickly added more complex diagnostic and treatment services and emerged as a new layer of provider within the health care hierarchy, taking their place between the smaller community hospital and the much more complex, university-based medical school hospitals. The components of this new layer of hospital service are referred to as "tertiary care medical centers." For the most part, these facilities were located in rural and far suburban areas. More specifically, they were far enough from city university hospitals to discourage local people from making the inconvenient trip to the city. In addition, costs for services at tertiary facilities were often less than at university-based hospitals. However, there also needed to be a critical mass of population in these "service areas" to support and generate the number of admissions per year necessary to keep a tertiary facility on firm financial ground. Many of these facilities had been established years earlier as small acute care hospitals, but because of a growing population and aggressive managerial foresight, over the years they added bed capacity and talented medical staff who could deliver more sophisticated medical services to the population, and hence they rapidly grew to become tertiary care of university-affiliated facilities.

The evolution of these local, community-based facilities into large tertiary care hospitals, along with the increased dependence on technology during the era between 1955 and 1970, also contributed to the decline of direct personal attention to patients. The cost of health care grew as additional funds were needed to make more services available and to purchase new technology. Many of these facilities were local community hospitals at heart, but because of their fortunate location, intelligent financial decisions, and a more aggressive mission, they attracted highly skilled and aggressive physicians which increased the facilities' reputations, which attracted patients from further distances.

Life became more complicated for these institutions, however. First, because of higher expectations on the part of physicians and patients, more and more money had to be earmarked for expansion and the newest and most sophisticated equipment. Second, because of the larger number of inpatients with increased acuity, referring physicians were not able to attend these patients around the clock, seven days a week. This created an interesting dilemma that was solved by affiliating with university hospitals that had large numbers of residents who were looking for a diversified training experience. This diversification was provided through affiliation agreements to send residents to the tertiary care facilities for rotations of duty. The university hospitals benefited because they could boast of well-developed and broad-based residency experience, which attracted the most talented people coming out of medical school. Universities could also increase their complement of residents, which made their programs even stronger. The tertiary hospital benefited because it now had a sufficient supply of skilled physicians to attend its patients around the clock when the private physicians were not available. The private physicians who were medical staff members at the tertiary hospitals benefited because the association with university hospitals kept them in touch with the newest diagnostic and treatment techniques. This also benefited the tertiary inpatient and reinforced the tertiary facility's reputation. In some instances, shared in-service programs benefited both institutions as well. It was not uncommon to see clinical services at the tertiary care hospitals compare very favorably with those at the university hospitals.

This was also a time when technology and specialization dominated care; there was a clear impact for the patient as well, but not, in all cases, for the better. Although the level of technology and expertise in diagnosis and treatment increased, individual attention given by their private physicians to patients' personal needs frequently decreased as more and more specialists from outside the local facility laid claim to patients. Although the concept of patient management had not yet been born, the problem demanding it certainly had been, and this helped to accelerate the decline in respect for physicians across the country. This decline continued more rapidly through the late 1960s, 1970s, and mid-1980s, when a displeased and more vocal patient population moved patient advocacy issues into the forefront.

GOVERNMENT GRABS HOLD

By the time Franklin Roosevelt's New Deal was in place, the federal government had a firm grip on hospitals. Direct control of finances and operations through government agencies were practically determining procedures and hospital operations. As government provided increased funding to hospitals, there were more and more strings attached. Restrictions on how many and which type of patients could be admitted, as well as which services could be provided, were imposed. In addition, state governments began to battle with the federal government for control over health care issues, with the conflicts depending on who perceived themselves to be the giver or taker or the winner or loser. To complicate things further, the Public Health Service began to make its influence felt with greater intensity. However, the biggest change was yet to come.

In 1965, President Johnson developed legislation that, when passed into law, inaugurated the age of Medicare and Medicaid. The provisions of this legislation would prove to be the most expensive form of government-funded medical care the country had seen.

STUDY QUESTIONS

1. Write a brief summary characterizing caregivers during the mid-1700s and early 1800s, and describe the facilities and techniques that were used for giving medical care. Address such issues as training, where services were provided, payment received for services, and level of expertise of providers.

2. How were almshouses of the early 1800s funded?

3. What factors facilitated local and federal government involvement in health care matters, and what were the arguments for and against this involvement?

4. Where was the first recognized hospital established in the United States, and what is its name today? Which prominent historical figure founded this hospital?

5. Briefly summarize the healing philosophies of the "regular" and the "mainline" medical groups, and give an example of treatment each group may have used.

6. Give two examples of how the military advanced medical education.

7. How did the rapid increase in industrialization affect the evolution of care during the 1800s?

8. When did specialization of medicine actually begin to appear? Name two of the earliest specialties that were established.

9. Explain why state and city governments were initially involved in regulating medical care, and what aspects of care local and federal government attempted to control.

10. Give an example of a major government program in the early 1900s that encouraged hospitals to provide medical care to the needy.

11. What element of health care did the Flexner Report address? What were some of its findings, and what institutions were affected?

Overview of Health Care Delivery in the United States

O B J E C T I V E S   F O R   S T U D Y

After reading this chapter, the student will

▶ Appreciate the major factors that drive the cost and scope of medical care services.

▶ Appreciate what aspects of our health care delivery system are affected by the federal government and how changes in legislation affect decision making and hospital strategic planning.

▶ Appreciate how payment to hospitals by third parties can affect the overall cost of medical care.

▶ Understand the complex economic and emotional factors that affect delivery and availability of health care service.

▶ Understand how the physician's role as provider and counsellor affects overall health care cost and demand.

▶ Understand how the hospital's role as a provider affects demand for service and the impact of this on overall health costs.

BASIC FACTORS THAT INFLUENCE THE ECONOMICS OF HEALTH CARE

The growth of the health care industry since 1950 has been especially dramatic, and much of the impetus for this growth lies in five fundamental elements:

- Entitlement to immediate access to health services
- Technology
- Legislation
- The payer system
- The aging and growing population

Entitlement Expectations

Entitlement expectations grow out of a long-standing belief that because this is a land of plenty, health care for Americans is an entitlement and should be available to the fullest extent possible to all. Although this ideal has not been fully realized to date, the principle of receiving virtually unlimited health care is strongly held by many Americans. This concept has encouraged the use of health care services to an extent unknown in other countries. It theoretically can lead to excessive use of health care services, and there are many today who strongly feel that such excess currently occurs. These feelings have led to simple questions that evoke complex answers: in what areas or services has excess been reached, and how are those areas identified and measured are just a few questions that barely scratch the surface of the problem of resource utilization in the health care industry.

Technology

Another of the significant elements that have encouraged utilization of health care and increased overall health care costs is the development and application of new technology. The advances in technology that we have seen over the last 40 years have been astonishing, admirable, extraordinarily beneficial, and expensive. We must understand, however, the distinction between the development of new technology and excesses regarding inappropriate application or utilization of that technology. Technology in itself is not the culprit because it has led to advances in medical care that have immeasurably improved the quality of all our lives and promises other improvements for the future. Researchers at medical centers working in conjunction with equipment manufacturers have produced equipment that has improved the chances for survival over illnesses that would have meant certain death only a few years ago. In other cases, technology has made the lives of millions of people more than tolerable, and still others lead lives filled with activity that could not have been expected only 5 or 10 years ago.

Radiology, for example, has seen some of the fastest growth in technology in all of medicine. As noted previously, however, these developments have not occurred without significant financial cost related to both research and implementation for routine clinical use. In fact, the HCFA (Health Care Finance Administration) estimates that health care research funding awarded to formalized investigation programs will equal approximately $19.9 billion in the year 2000. Some university-based hospitals may receive at least $20 million a year in grant money to support multiple research projects of 1 to 5 years duration. Twenty years ago, the most expensive diagnostic X-ray machines would have cost about $500,000. We now purchase magnetic resonance (MR) and computed tomography scanners that cost over $1.3 million. In the case of MR equipment, additional expenditures of up to $500,000 are necessary to provide a proper site for the device. In addition to these up-front acquisition costs, most of these hi-tech devices demand service contracts that can cost $120,000 per year per machine, so one-time purchase costs are not the only problem. Once these machines are operating, expenses increase. Table 2-1 shows the rate of inflation for health care over a number of years.

The enthusiasm for new technology was encouraged by claims of advanced diagnostic capabilities. Claims of improved diagnostic accuracy, shorter examination time (greater efficiency), or exaggerated capabilities for diagnosing diseases were used as strong selling points. Another rationale used to encourage the purchase of new technology was savings—it promised to permit the physician to obtain the same or higher-quality diagnosis previously obtained by other, multiple conventional tests. In other words, one expensive piece of equipment would reduce costs because multiple studies could be avoided.

Unfortunately, in some cases the performance of many of these machines fell short of overly enthusiastic clinical and operational benefits. Once they were in place, there was immediate pressure to increase their utilization to justify their expense, and this also contributed to the overall health care bill. Today, the technology race continues; however, both researchers and manufacturers view the development of future products with much more financial scrutiny and realism than in the past. Hospital administrators base purchases on more substantial criteria as well. We should never try to stop the development of new technology, but we must apply a higher level of wisdom in its development, application, and utility.

Another way in which new technology has affected overall health care should be considered. New technology has always been used as a marketing tool by its owners. Health care providers point with pride to their inclusion on the list of those who offer "leading edge" or "state-of-the-art" technology, and patients are justifiably attracted to new technology and gain confidence when diagnosed or treated by what is perceived to be the most advanced device available. In addition, administrators have learned from hard experience that one of the surest ways to attract talented physicians to their staffs as well as to maintain professional interest among technologists and incumbent physicians is to promise and have the latest equipment available for use. Attracting talented physicians is important for hospitals because of the referrals highly skilled physicians can generate for both outpatient and inpatient admissions. This is particularly true at tertiary and university-based hospitals.

Litigation

Another element that has pushed the growth of health care expenses is the extremely high rate and size of awards given through litigation against facilities and practitioners. The United States is the highest-ranking country in both the frequency of health care litigation and the size of awards given to plaintiffs. Table 2-2 shows awards over time. The right to take legal action against health care institutions and practitioners is considered by many health care economists to be a significant contributor to increased utilization of health care services because physicians fearing litigation may order unnecessary diagnostic tests and overly aggressive treatments for their patients.

As the social atmosphere encourages and even promotes legal action, liability insurance premiums charged to physicians and facilities increase. This cost is rolled into the overall expense of providing health care and is reflected in higher group health insurance premiums as well as in the Medicare/Medicaid taxes that we all pay. There is the potential that malpractice litigation has given some physicians a basis for ordering unnecessary tests under the banner of medicolegal threats.

(Text continues on page 36)

▶ TABLE 2-1
NATIONAL HEALTH EXPENDITURES: 1960 TO 1993 (INCLUDES PUERTO RICO AND OUTLYING AREAS)

	TOTAL[1]			Health Services and Supplies					Public		
					Private					Medical payments	
					Out-of-pocket payments						
YEAR	Total (bil. dol.)	Per capita (dol.)	Percent of GDP[2]	Total[3] (bil. dol.)	Total (bil. dol.)	Percent of total private	Insurance premiums (bil. dol.)	Total (bil. dol.)	Medicare (bil. dol.)	Public assistance (bil. dol.)
1960	27.1	143	5.3	19.8	13.4	67.5	5.9	5.7	—	0.5
1965	41.6	204	5.9	29.9	19.0	63.6	10.0	8.3	—	1.7
1970	74.3	346	7.4	44.0	25.4	57.7	16.9	25.0	7.7	6.3
1971	82.2	379	7.5	48.1	26.9	55.9	19.2	28.2	8.5	7.7
1972	92.3	421	7.7	53.9	29.6	55.0	22.0	31.8	9.4	8.9
1973	102.4	464	7.6	59.7	32.6	54.5	24.8	35.9	10.8	10.2
1974	115.9	521	7.9	65.9	35.8	54.3	27.5	42.8	13.5	11.9
1975	132.6	591	8.4	74.1	39.1	52.8	32.0	50.2	16.4	14.5
1976	151.9	671	8.6	85.7	43.2	50.4	38.5	56.9	19.8	16.4
1977	172.6	755	8.7	98.6	47.5	48.2	46.7	64.7	23.0	18.8
1978	193.2	838	8.7	109.7	51.0	46.5	53.6	73.6	26.8	20.9

1979	218.3	937	8.8	124.0	55.9	45.1	62.2	84.0	31.0	23.9
1980	251.1	1,068	9.3	141.3	61.3	43.4	72.1	98.1	37.5	28.0
1981	291.4	1,227	9.6	164.3	69.6	42.4	85.1	113.9	44.9	32.6
1982	328.2	1,369	10.4	186.5	76.5	41.0	99.1	126.9	52.5	34.6
1983	360.8	1,490	10.6	205.3	83.0	40.4	110.6	139.5	59.8	38.0
1984	396.0	1,620	10.5	228.0	90.4	39.6	125.1	151.6	66.5	41.1
1985	434.5	1,761	10.8	252.9	98.8	39.1	139.8	165.2	72.2	44.5
1986	466.0	1,871	10.9	268.7	105.0	39.1	147.8	180.4	76.9	49.0
1987	506.2	2,013	11.1	291.3	111.6	38.3	162.3	196.6	82.3	54.0
1988	562.3	2,214	11.5	327.5	123.0	37.6	184.8	213.7	89.4	58.8
1989	623.9	2,433	11.9	361.7	127.8	35.3	211.7	240.1	102.6	66.4
1990	696.6	2,686	12.6	399.8	138.3	34.6	236.9	272.5	112.1	80.5
1991	755.6	2,882	13.2	422.8	143.3	33.9	252.8	308.0	123.3	99.1
1992	820.3	3,094	13.6	451.7	150.6	33.3	272.7	341.2	138.3	113.5
1993	884.2	3,299	13.9	484.3	157.5	32.5	296.1	370.9	154.2	122.9

— Represents zero. [1]Includes medical research and medical facilities construction.
[2]GDP = Gross domestic product.
[3]Includes other sources of funds not shown separately.
(Source: U.S. Health Care Financing Administration, *Health Care Financing Review*, Winter 1994)

Shows the cost of health care over several decades from several perspectives. The continued increase of both state and federal dollars spent on health care has the same effect on our economy as does increasing national debt. If such inflation continues, the government will not have enough money to cover future health care costs.

▶ TABLE 2–2

A. SUMMARY ANALYSIS
ALL VERDICTS
HOSPITAL & PHYSICIAN CASES COMBINED

YEAR	FULL RANGE OF VERDICTS	AVERAGE VERDICT
1988	$852,000 to $2,300	$300,000
1991	$1,250,000 to $145,000	$465,000

Plaintiff Recoverage Rate Is Approximately 39%

B. SUMMARY OF SELECTED CATEGORIES
MALPRACTICE
HOSPITAL & PHYSICIAN CASES COMBINED

	WRONGFUL DEATH			MALPRACTICE, DIAGNOSIS		
	Probability Range	Average Verdict	Verdict Range	Probability Range	Average Verdict	Verdict Range
1988	$185,000 to $565,017	$372,000	$10,000 to $22,000,000	$200,000 to $680,000	$500,000	$2,000 to $3,020,000
1991	$409,360 to $972,000	$602,000	$75,000 to $8,100,000	$153,000 to $1,160,000	$856,250	$90,000 to $2,260,000

Average Plaintiff Recovery Rate = 40%

Average Time Needed from Date of Injury to Verdict, 61 Months
Average Time Needed from Filing to Verdict, 41 Months

C. SUMMARY OF SELECTED CATEGORIES
MALPRACTICE, SELECTED CATEGORIES
PHYSICIAN CASES
1991

	WRONGFUL DEATH			MALPRACTICE, DIAGNOSIS			NEGLIGENT SUPERVISION		
	Probability Range	Average Verdict	Verdict Range	Probability Range	Average Verdict	Verdict Range	Probability Range	Average Verdict	Verdict Range
Physicians	$296,655 to $1,000,000	$500,000	$50,000 to $5,700,000	$217,000 to $1,250,000	$500,000	$22,000 to $4,619,914	—	—	—
Average Plaintiff Recovery Rate	38%								
Hospitals	$1,300,000 to $2,700,000	$653,000	$102,000 to $4,450,000	$204,000 to $1,449,160	$500,000	$10,000 to $26,000,000	$48,488 to $583,000	$250,000	$12,750 to $6,500,000
Average Plaintiff Recovery Rate	53%								

Malpractice, Diagnosis: Includes improper or delayed evaluations leading to loss of life, and actions that prevented prompt treatment or caused the loss of limbs, emotional distress, or permanant injury.
Wrongful Death: Includes improper diagnosis, inadequate treatment, inappropriate medication.
Negligent Supervision: Includes failure to attend to the patient's safety needs such as claims relating to poor observation.
(Source: *Trends in Health Care Provider Liability: An Analysis of Jury Verdicts.* Copyright 1992 by LRP Publications, Horsham, PA. 19044-0980. All rights reserved.)

Shows selected elements of litigation. These figures indicate the size of settlements that have become common today. Settlements such as these influence the degree of risk physicians are willing to take when considering the type and number of tests to order for their patients. They also significantly affect the cost of liability insurance coverage for both hospitals and physicians.

The bulk of malpractice claims are actually against a relatively small number of the nation's physicians, as described in a study done by Rolph in 1981. In a group of 8000 insured physicians, 10% of all claims were against 0.6% of all licensed physicians. Attorneys are also considered by some to be driving the high rate of litigation. In some states, their fees for obtaining favorable judgments have been as high as 40%. These fees, however, have been reduced by recent legislation, and the role of attorneys is considered by some researchers, such as Phelps, to be "Less of an engine to increasing malpractice judgments than has been thought." Phelps does point out that the presence of malpractice insurance subscriptions by physicians does much more to encourage malpractice claims. He further states that only approximately 1 in 15 to 1 in 25 negligently injured people actually receive compensation.

The Payer System

Payer systems of the past have also contributed to the rapid acceleration of costs for diagnostic tests, treatment, and related services. The late 1950s saw some new and important changes in the federal government's willingness to affect or control our health care delivery system, principally evidenced by a growing number of laws that reflected strong public sentiment about entitlement to services. As noted earlier in this chapter, as new technology and treatments were developed and publicized at an accelerated rate, more people wanted access and pressed for government to get involved on their behalf. As the entitlement philosophy increased throughout the country in strength, the utilization of health care services began to increase substantially, leading directly to the Social Security Act of 1964, which brought about Medicare and Medicaid.

Under this law, hospitals would be paid for the services they provided to patients who were at least 65 years of age and met other Medicare benefits criteria. In addition, under the Social Security Act, each state had to develop a plan to provide health care services for a large group of people who could not pay out of pocket for health care services. The state plan was called Medicaid. The Medicare and Medicaid programs seemed to validate entitlement to services. An interesting aspect of our health care delivery system is that payment for services is the responsibility of someone other than the patient. In fact, the federal government pays approximately 55% of the total health care bill through Medicare and supplements to Medicaid. Medicare and Medicaid payments were to be in part paid by surplus Social Security funds. Much of the balance of the nation's health care expenses was covered by Blue Cross and Blue Shield and by for-profit companies such as Prudential, Metropolitan, and Aetna. The point to appreciate here is that under a system in which predominantly a "third party," that is, an insurance group and the government, covered a bill based on accumulated costs that were recommended and generated by the provider, there was little incentive for either the patient, the physician, or the facility to attempt to hold back on services or cost per service. This was especially true when the physician and facility generated revenue from the services they provided.

In this perceived "no pay" environment, utilization of services accelerated significantly. In fact, from 1982 to 1992, use of staffed beds changed considerably (Table 2-3). In 1989, medical equipment sales totaled $13.5 billion. In 1990, all of these factors generated a need for $10 billion in new construction for new or expanded health care services. This generated a *need* for increased employment as well. You will see later in this text there is a strong relationship between capital expenditures and operating expenses. In 1991, more than 4.3 million people were employed in direct patient care occupations, and the Bureau of Labor and Statistics projected that future employment in health care will reach 12.9 million by the year 2005.

Aging Population

The increasing age of the U.S. population has made an impact on the overall needs for health care services and their related costs; Table 2-4 shows this in specific terms. As you will see, the average age of our population in 2005 is expected to be substantially higher than at present.

THE RETROSPECTIVE REIMBURSEMENT/PAYMENT SYSTEM

It will be of value to describe briefly the payment system that resulted from the Medicare legislation. Retrospective in this sense means that the third party payer paid (reimbursed) the hospital after services were rendered and after costs were tabulated. Because of this third-party retrospective reimbursement system, there was a growing feeling through the 1970s that there may indeed be a "free lunch" at the health care table where providers were almost encouraged to provide more and more services. These services would generate more revenue for providers while many patients could receive services without significant out-of-pocket expenses. To meet this growing demand for services produced by more physicians, new and more complex treatments were devised. In addition, the rapid growth of new technology answered the need for new and more sophisticated diagnostic capabilities.

Indeed, the "retrospective reimbursement" system encouraged this acceleration in activity because payment to hospitals was based on the operating costs that were generated during the patient's stay. As hospitals performed more tests and services, operating costs increased and reimbursement was increased accordingly, leading to dramatic increases in expenses for additional equipment and personnel. Thus, each year the reimbursement system reassured health care administrators, patients, and physicians that if their costs increased, funds would be available to cover them. This made it relatively easy to acquire new equipment, more buildings, new services, and additional personnel. Physicians were able to encourage hospital administrators to buy new and more expensive equipment as well as to improve existing facilities because the incremental costs would be largely covered by the federal government, Blue Cross, or private insurance companies. Table 2-5 shows hospital admissions from 1982 to 1992.

IMPLEMENTATION OF THE PROSPECTIVE PAYMENT SYSTEM

At first, health care administrators were skeptical of the retrospective Medicare and Medicaid system; however, it proved to be a boon to the growth of the industry—so much so that after 10 years of almost unchecked inflation, there was significant sentiment to overhaul or do away with the retrospective payment system (Fig. 2-1). In 1980, the Reagan Administration promoted and signed into law the nation's prospective payment system, which promised to change this cycle of spend-and-reimburse substantially. Figure 2-2 shows the cost of health care relative to the country's gross national product (GNP).

These basic elements created a complex matrix of ironies. On the one hand, there was the need continually to improve the well-established higher level of care that had been fostered and encouraged by retrospective reimbursement. On the other hand, the activity and demand for services this philosophy encouraged became too expensive for the national budget. In fact, the huge increases in health care spending began to pose a potentially catastrophic threat to the country's economy. By the late 1970s and early 1980s, we were beginning to realize as a nation that there is, after all, no free lunch at the health care table.

(*Text continues on page 43*)

▶ TABLE 2-3
A. DISTRIBUTION OF COMMUNITY HOSPITALS, BY BED-SIZE, 1982 AND 1991–1992

	NUMBER OF HOSPITALS			PERCENT CHANGE	
	1982	1991	1992	1982–1992	1991–1992
Total community hospitals	5,801	5,342	5,292	−8.8%	−0.9
Urban community hospitals	3,041	2,921	3,007	−1.1%	2.9
6–24 Beds	43	36	39	−9.3%	8.3
25–49	208	174	197	−5.3%	13.2
50–99	463	440	470	1.5%	6.8
100–199	766	791	823	7.4%	4.0
200–299	590	617	612	3.7%	−0.8
300–399	379	369	382	0.8%	3.5
400–499	265	218	195	−26.4%	−10.6
500 or more	327	276	289	−11.6%	4.7
Rural community hospitals	2,760	2,421	2,285	−17.2%	−5.6
6–24 Beds	192	186	191	−0.5%	2.7
25–49	772	748	703	−8.9%	−6.0
50–99	977	804	740	−24.3%	−8.0
100–199	614	520	498	−18.9%	−4.2
200–299	148	124	113	−23.6%	−8.9
300–399	44	29	30	−31.8%	3.4
400–499	8	5	6	−25.0%	20.0
500 or more	5	5	4	−20.0%	−20.0

(Source: *AHA Hospital Statistics, 1993 Edition.* Copyright by the American Hospital Association.)

B. EMPLOYMENT IN THE HEALTH SERVICE INDUSTRIES: 1980 TO 1994 (IN THOUSANDS)

INDUSTRY	1987 SIC CODE[1]	1980	1985	1990	1992	1993	1994
Health services[2]	80	5,278	6,293	7,814	8,490	8,767	9,032
Offices and clinics of MDs	801	802	1,028	1,338	1,463	1,512	1,562
Offices and clinics of dentists	802	(NA)	439	513	541	560	590
Offices and clinics of other practitioners	804	96	165	277	327	356	389
Nursing and personal care facilities	805	997	1,198	1,415	1,533	1,580	1,633
Skilled nursing care facilities	8051	(NA)	791	989	1,094	1,130	1,170
Intermediate care facilities	8052	(NA)	(NA)	200	217	222	229
Other, n.e.c.[3]	8059	(NA)	(NA)	227	222	228	233
Hospitals	806	2,750	2,997	3,549	3,750	3,787	3,790
General medical and surgical hospitals	8062	(NA)	2,811	3,268	3,449	3,485	3,492
Psychiatric hospitals	8063	(NA)	59	104	102	97	94
Specialty hospitals, except psychiatric	8069	(NA)	126	176	199	205	204
Medical and dental laboratories	807	105	119	166	180	190	202
Home health care services	808	(NA)	152	291	398	462	533

NA Not available. [1]Based on the 1987 Standard Industrial Classification code; see text, section 13. [2]Includes other industries not shown separately. [3]N.e.c. means not elsewhere classified.
(Source: U.S. Bureau of Labor Statistics, *Bulletin 2445*, and *Employment and Earnings*, monthly, March and June issues.)

Shows the distribution of hospitals with various bed capacities in the United States. Because many hospitals' occupancy rates have fallen substantially over the last five years, judging hospital size by licensed bed capacity may be misleading. It is not unusual to see occupancy at 50% to 60% of total licensed beds.

▶ TABLE 2–4
POPULATION 65 YEARS OLD AND OVER, BY AGE GROUP AND SEX, 1980 TO 1991, AND PROJECTIONS, 2000 (AS OF APRIL, EXCEPT 1991 AND 2000, AS OF JULY. PROJECTION BASED ON MIDDLE SERIES)

AGE GROUP AND SEX	NUMBER (1,000)				PERCENT DISTRIBUTION			
	1980	1990	1991	2000, projected	1980	1990	1991	2000, projected
Persons 65 yrs. and over	25,549	31,079	31,754	34,886	100.0	100.0	100.0	100.0
65 to 69 years old	8,782	10,066	10,037	9,469	34.3	32.4	31.6	27.1
70 to 74 years old	6,796	7,980	8,242	8,789	26.6	25.7	26.0	25.2
75 to 79 years old	4,794	6,103	6,279	7,447	18.8	19.6	19.8	21.3
80 to 84 years old	2,935	3,909	4,035	4,892	11.5	12.6	12.7	14.0
85 years old and over	2,240	3,021	3,160	4,289	8.8	9.7	10.0	12.3
Males, 65 years and over	10,305	12,493	12,791	14,402	100.0	100.0	100.0	100.0
65 to 69 years old	3,303	4,508	4,491	4,369	37.8	36.1	35.1	30.3
70 to 74 years old	2,854	3,399	3,531	3,911	27.7	27.2	27.6	27.2
75 to 79 years old	1,848	2,389	2,482	3,100	18.0	19.1	19.4	21.5
80 to 84 years old	1,019	1,356	1,406	1,807	9.9	10.9	11.0	12.5
85 years old and over	682	841	881	1,215	6.6	6.7	6.9	8.4
Females, 65 years and over	15,245	18,586	18,962	20,484	100.0	100.0	100.0	100.0
65 to 69 years old	4,880	5,558	5,546	5,100	31.9	29.9	29.2	24.9
70 to 74 years old	3,945	4,580	4,712	4,878	25.9	24.6	24.6	23.8
75 to 79 years old	2,846	3,714	3,797	4,347	19.3	20.0	20.0	21.2
80 to 84 years old	1,916	2,553	2,629	3,086	12.6	13.7	13.9	15.1
85 years old and over	1,559	2,180	2,279	3,074	10.3	11.7	12.0	15.0

(Source: U.S. Bureau of the Census, *Current Population Reports*, P25-1092 and P25-1095.)

Shows the changing mix of population demographics in the U.S. This has clear implications for future health care costs per capita and for the nature of services that will be needed.

A. SELECTED MEASURES IN COMMUNITY HOSPITALS, 1984 AND 1993–94

MEASURE	YEAR			PERCENT CHANGE[1]	
	1984	1994	1993	1984–94	1993–94
Hospitals	5,759	5,229	5,261	−9.2%	−0.6%
Beds (000s)	1,017	902	919	−11.3%	−1.8%
Average number of beds per hospital	177	173	175	−2.3%	−1.1%
Admissions (000s)	35,155	30,718	30,748	−12.6%	−0.1%
Average daily census (000s)	702	568	592	−19.1%	−4.0%
Average length of stay, days	7.3	6.7	7.0	−8.2%	−4.3%
Inpatient days (000s)	256,603	207,180	215,889	−19.3%	−4.0%
Surgical operations (000s)	19,908	22,988	22,806	15.5%	0.8%
Bassinets (000s)[2]	75	66	66	−13.0%	−0.4%
Births (000s)[2]	3,456	3,809	3,807	10.2%	0.1%
Outpatient visits (000s)[3]	211,961	382,924	366,885	80.7%	4.4%

[1]Percent changes are based on actual figures, not rounded.
[2]Based only on hospitals reporting newborn data.
[3]Based only on hospitals reporting outpatient visits.
(Source: *AHA Hospital Statistics, 1993 Edition.* Copyright by the American Hospital Association.)

continued

B. HOSPITAL USE RATES, BY TYPE OF HOSPITAL: 1972 TO 1991 [SEE ALSO *HISTORICAL STATISTICS, COLONIAL TIMES TO 1970*, SERIES B 364-367]

TYPE OF HOSPITAL	1972	1980	1985	1986	1987	1988	1989	1990	1991	1993
Community hospitals:										
Admissions per 1,000 population[1]	147	159	141	135	130	129	126	125	123	119
Admissions per bed	35	37	33	33	33	33	33	34	34	33
Average length of stay[2] (days)	7.9	7.6	7.1	7.1	7.2	7.2	7.2	7.2	7.3	7.0
Outpatient visits per admission	1.8	5.6	6.5	7.2	7.8	8.6	9.2	9.7	10.4	11.9
Outpatient visits per 1,000 population[1]	777	890	919	966	1,013	1,101	1,158	1,206	1,277	1,423
Surgical operations (million)	14.8	18.8	20.1	20.5	20.8	21.4	21.3	21.9	22.4	22.8
Number per admission	0.5	0.5	0.6	0.6	0.7	0.7	0.7	0.7	0.7	0.7
Non-Federal psychiatric:										
Admissions per 1,000 population[1]	2.8	2.5	2.5	2.5	2.6	2.8	2.9	2.9	2.9	2.9
Days in hospital per 1,000 population[1]	661	295	224	217	214	209	201	190	179	149

[1]Based on Bureau of the Census estimated resident population as of July 1. Estimates reflect revisions based on the 1990 Census of Population.
[2]Number of inpatient days divided by number of admissions. (Source: *AHA Hospital Statistics, 1993 Edition* (copyright by the American Hospital Association); and unpublished data.)

Shows declining number of admissions as more procedures and tests are performed on an outpatient basis. This trend now seen along the East Coast is expected to continue over the next two to four years until it reaches levels that have already been reached along the West Coast and in many Midwestern states.

Retrospective Payment System

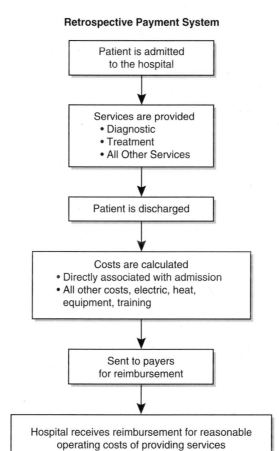

Patient is admitted
to the hospital

↓

Services are provided
• Diagnostic
• Treatment
• All Other Services

↓

Patient is discharged

↓

Costs are calculated
• Directly associated with admission
• All other costs, electric, heat,
  equipment, training

↓

Sent to payers
for reimbursement

↓

Hospital receives reimbursement for reasonable
operating costs of providing services

▶ **FIGURE 2-1** Payment through the retrospective system encouraged added services and costs because hospitals received reimbursement based on the operating and capital costs generated by these services.

The new resolve demonstrated by the proposal of prospective payment was the first major signal that federal legislators had their financial backs to the wall: The rapidly expanding bite of health care was taking out of GNP had to be brought under control.

THE COMPLEXITY OF THE HEALTH CARE SYSTEM

The first significant salvo of cost cutting came at a time when increased awareness on the part of patients was producing a demand for higher-quality services. The dilemma inherent in establishing new criteria for meeting these increased demands at a time when reimbursement for services is dramatically reduced represents the fundamental challenge facing all health care providers today: to deliver higher-quality health care at prices the country can afford. Another perplexing factor now is the sheer size of the industry and the effect cost cutting has on the general economy with respect to jobs (Table 2-6).

Government Health Expenditures as a Percent of Total Government Expenditures: Selected Years 1960–93		
Year	Federal Expenditures	State and Local Expenditures
	Percent	
1960	3.1	7.8
1965	3.9	7.6
1966	5.2	7.5
1967	7.3	7.6
1970	8.5	7.8
1975	10.0	8.5
1980	11.7	9.9
1985	12.7	11.0
1990	15.4	12.9
1991	16.9	12.8
1992	17.4	12.6
1993	18.6	12.4

▶ **FIGURE 2–2** Shows expansion of health care expenses as a percentage of GNP. The GNP is used as a standard because it is the value of all goods and services produced in the United States. (Sources: Health Care Financing Administration. Office of the Actuary: Data from the Office of National Health Statistics; and the U.S. Department of Commerce, Bureau of Economic Analysis.)

The health care industry in 1995 was projected by HCFA to represent 14.2% of the GNP, or $1 trillion. The rapid rise in the percentage of the GNP taken up by health costs is shown below and hospital services specifically account for slightly more than one third of these expenses. However, there are signs that the rate of annual increase that has become so alarming is beginning to cool in recent years to less than 8%.

Typically, when we think of health care, we primarily consider physicians, hospitals, nursing homes, and private offices (Table 2-7A, B). Although hospital costs account for the largest portion of the overall cost of health care, we must also consider the many industries that also are a part of the health care industry. These industries, to name just a few, include X-ray equipment and film manufacturers, surgical instrument suppliers and manufacturers, wheelchair manufacturers, pharmaceutical companies, and insurance companies.

Another link in the health care food chain is the huge contingent of federal and state regulatory agencies, which employ hundreds of thousands of people. Consider further the many people who are employed by the legal industry whose work depends on the health care delivery system. To broaden the range one step further, we can also consider the fairly significant portion of the construction industry, comprising architects, design engineers, and construction workers, who build and renovate medical facilities. During 1990, more than $10 billion was spent on building and renovation projects associated with health care facilities. Medical insurance companies are another large health care-related industry that employs hundreds of thousands of people.

(*Text continues on page 50*)

▶ TABLE 2–6
GROSS NATIONAL PRODUCT IN DOMESTIC TRADE AND SERVICE INDUSTRIES IN CURRENT AND CONSTANT (1982) DOLLARS: 1980 TO 1992
[IN BILLIONS OF DOLLARS, EXCEPT PERCENT. BASED ON 1972 STANDARD INDUSTRIAL CLASSIFICATION]

INDUSTRY	CURRENT DOLLARS				CONSTANT (1982) DOLLARS					
	1980	1985	1988	1989	1980	1985	1988	1989	1992	CURRENT
Wholesale and retail trade	436.8	658.2	777.3	825.4	481.8	621.5	689.8	716.6	827.6	
Percent of gross national product	16.1	16.4	15.9	15.9	15.1	17.2	17.2	17.4	16.6	
Wholesale trade	193.9	280.8	317.4	339.5	200.1	267.1	290.6	304.7	340.9	
Retail trade	245.0	377.4	459.9	486.0	281.7	354.4	399.2	412.0	486.7	
Services	374.0	648.1	885.2	970.5	450.9	538.6	623.3	652.3	889.9	1,182.7
Percent of gross national product	13.7	16.1	18.2	18.7	14.1	14.9	15.5	15.8	17.9	19.6
Hotels and other lodging places	18.9	30.4	41.2	44.5	22.3	26.0	31.2	32.5	30.4	53.9
Personal services	18.8	29.7	38.5	43.0	22.3	25.2	28.6	30.3	30.4	39.0
Business services	68.8	145.8	202.1	222.9	83.9	120.8	147.7	158.7	173.7	220.5
Auto repair, services, and garages	21.1	33.2	40.5	43.6	24.8	28.7	28.3	28.8	37.1	48.8
Miscellaneous repair services	9.2	12.4	15.6	16.9	10.6	10.7	11.7	12.2	13.9	16.9
Motion pictures	5.0	9.0	13.5	14.7	5.7	7.5	9.5	9.8	14.6	19.3
Amusement and recreation services	12.4	19.9	27.4	29.8	13.4	17.5	21.8	22.8	40.8	51.1
Health services	108.1	184.6	250.3	273.3	133.8	148.6	161.1	164.4	252.0	364.4
Legal services	23.3	46.3	68.7	75.2	30.6	33.5	40.6	41.8	66.0	88.7
Educational services	16.0	25.8	32.5	35.5	18.9	22.1	23.3	24.1	35.1	45.6
Social services, membership organizations	26.3	38.3	51.2	56.0	30.2	33.3	39.0	40.9	59.6	70.2
Miscellaneous professional services	39.6	63.6	93.9	104.9	47.0	56.0	71.3	76.4	112.2	154.1
Private households	6.6	9.0	9.7	10.3	7.4	8.8	9.2	9.5	8.8	10.1

(Source: U.S. Health Care Financing Administration, *Health Care Review.*)

Shows values of goods and services produced by major industries, including health care. Note how the health care figures escalated during the 1980s. This escalation actually began in the mid-1960s and caused sufficient alarm in Washington and among business owners that it elicited the response of the prospective payment model.

▶ TABLE 2-7
A. NATIONAL HEALTH EXPENDITURES, BY TYPE OF SERVICE AGGREGATE AMOUNT AND AVERAGE ANNUAL CHANGE (CALENDAR YEARS 1980–2005)

	1980	1990	1991	1992	1993	1994	1995	2000	2005
							PROJECTED		
					Aggregate amount (billions)				
National Health Expenditures	$251.1	$696.6	$755.6	$820.3	$884.2	$938.3	$1,007.6	$1,481.7	$2,173.7
Personal health care	220.1	612.4	670.8	729.7	782.5	832.5	897.7	1,334.3	1,973.4
Hospital care	102.7	256.5	282.3	306.0	326.6	341.7	364.5	518.3	736.8
Physician services	45.2	140.5	150.3	161.8	171.2	182.7	198.0	309.8	483.6
Dental services	13.3	30.4	31.7	34.7	37.4	40.0	42.9	59.1	79.1
Other professional services	6.4	36.0	40.4	46.4	51.2	56.7	62.9	103.3	166.4
Home health care	1.9	11.1	13.2	16.8	20.8	24.2	27.9	45.9	68.0
Drugs and other medical non-durables	21.6	61.2	67.1	70.8	75.0	79.0	84.7	122.3	178.6
Vision products and other medical durables	4.5	10.5	11.3	12.0	12.6	13.2	13.9	17.9	22.6
Nursing home care	20.5	54.8	60.8	65.5	69.6	74.2	80.2	121.2	179.6
Other personal health care	4.0	11.4	13.6	15.8	18.2	20.9	22.7	36.5	58.7
Program administration and net cost of private health insurance	12.1	38.3	37.0	39.5	48.0	50.3	51.9	74.1	107.3
Government public health activities	7.2	21.6	22.9	23.7	24.7	26.1	27.9	37.2	48.6
Research	5.5	12.2	12.9	14.2	14.4	15.4	15.9	19.6	24.4
Construction	6.2	12.1	11.9	13.2	14.6	14.1	14.2	16.5	20.0

Average annual percent change from previous year shown

National Health Expenditures	10.7%	8.5%	8.6%	7.8%	6.1%	7.4%	8.0%	8.0%
Personal health care	10.8	9.5	8.8	7.2	6.4	7.8	8.2	8.1
Hospital care	9.6	10.0	8.4	6.7	4.6	6.7	7.3	7.3
Physician services	12.0	7.0	7.6	5.8	6.7	8.4	9.4	9.3
Dental services	8.6	4.2	.6	7.7	7.0	7.2	6.6	6.0
Other professional services	18.9	12.3	14.8	10.4	10.6	11.0	10.4	10.0
Home health care	19.4	19.2	27.4	23.8	16.2	15.5	10.5	8.2
Drugs and other medical non-durables	11.0	9.5	5.5	5.9	5.4	7.1	7.6	7.9
Vision products and other medical durables	8.9	7.2	6.4	5.3	4.3	5.5	5.1	4.8
Nursing home care	10.3	10.9	7.8	6.3	6.6	8.0	8.6	8.2
Other personal health care	11.0	21.4	14.4	15.0	15.0	8.7	10.0	10.0
Program administration and net cost of private health insurance	12.2	−3.3	6.6	21.5	4.8	3.2	7.4	7.7
Government public health activities	11.5	6.4	3.4	4.2	5.6	6.9	5.9	5.5
Research	8.4	5.6	10.3	1.1	6.8	3.5	4.3	4.5
Construction	7.0	−1.9	11.4	10.8	−3.4	0.5	3.0	4.0

NOTE: Numbers and percents may not add to total because of rounding.

continued

▲ TABLE 2–7 *Continued*

B. HOSPITAL CARE EXPENDITURES AGGREGATE AND PER CAPITA AMOUNTS AND PERCENT DISTRIBUTION, BY SOURCE OF FUNDS (SELECTED YEARS 1960–93)

| | | | THIRD-PARTY PAYMENTS | | | | | | | |
| | | Out-of-Pocket | | Private Health | Other Private | | Government | | | |
Year	Total	Payments	Total	Insurance	Funds	Total	Federal	State and Local	Medicare[1]	Medicaid[2]
					Amount in Billions					
1960	$9.3	$1.9	$7.4	$3.3	$0.1	$3.9	$1.6	$2.3	—	—
1970	28.0	2.5	25.5	9.6	0.9	15.0	9.9	5.1	$5.3	$2.2
1980	102.7	5.3	97.4	38.7	5.0	53.7	40.9	12.8	26.3	8.5
1985	168.2	8.8	159.4	61.0	8.3	90.1	71.1	19.0	48.9	13.7
1987	194.1	8.7	185.4	72.2	9.8	103.5	78.7	24.8	53.0	16.6
1989	231.8	9.7	222.2	88.1	12.4	121.7	93.0	28.7	62.8	20.9
1990	256.5	9.8	246.8	95.7	13.8	137.3	103.4	33.9	68.5	26.5
1991	282.3	9.6	272.7	102.8	15.1	154.8	120.3	34.5	74.9	34.5
1992	306.0	9.0	297.0	109.1	15.9	172.0	137.3	34.7	84.2	41.0
1993	326.6	9.1	317.4	117.8	16.8	182.9	149.2	33.7	92.7	42.4

Per Capita Amount

Year										
1960	$49	$10	$39	$17	$21	$1	$8	$12	—	—
1970	130	12	119	45	70	4	46	24	(3)	(3)
1980	437	23	414	165	228	21	174	55	(3)	(3)
1985	682	36	646	247	365	34	288	77	(3)	(3)
1987	772	35	737	287	411	39	313	99	(3)	(3)
1989	904	38	866	344	475	48	363	112	(3)	(3)
1990	989	38	951	369	530	53	399	131	(3)	(3)
1991	1,077	37	1,040	392	591	57	459	132	(3)	(3)
1992	1,154	34	1,120	412	649	60	518	131	(3)	(3)
1993	1,218	34	1,184	439	682	63	557	126	(3)	(3)

Percent Distribution

Year										
1960	100.0	20.7	79.3	35.6	42.5	1.2	17.3	25.2	—	—
1970	100.0	9.0	91.0	34.3	53.5	3.2	35.2	18.2	18.8	8.0
1980	100.0	5.2	94.8	37.7	52.3	4.9	39.8	12.5	25.6	8.3
1985	100.0	5.2	94.8	36.3	53.6	4.9	42.3	11.3	29.1	8.1
1987	100.0	4.5	95.5	37.2	53.3	5.0	40.5	12.8	27.3	8.5
1989	100.0	4.2	95.8	38.0	52.5	5.3	40.1	12.4	27.1	9.0
1990	100.0	3.8	96.2	37.3	53.5	5.4	40.3	13.2	26.7	10.3
1991	100.0	3.4	96.6	36.4	54.8	5.3	42.6	12.2	26.5	12.2
1992	100.0	2.9	97.1	35.7	56.2	5.2	44.9	11.3	27.5	13.4
1993	100.0	2.8	97.2	36.1	56.0	5.2	45.7	10.3	28.4	13.0

1 Subset of Federal funds.

2 Subset of Federal and State and local funds.

(3) Calculation of per capita estimates is inappropriate.

NOTES: Per capita amounts based on July 1 Social Security area population estimates for each year, 1960–90. 1991–93 estimated by the Health Care Financing Administration. Numbers and percents may not add to totals because of rounding.

(Source: Health Care Financing Administration, Office of the Actuary.)

Shows the distribution of health care expenses within the industry.

Prospective Payment Under DRG

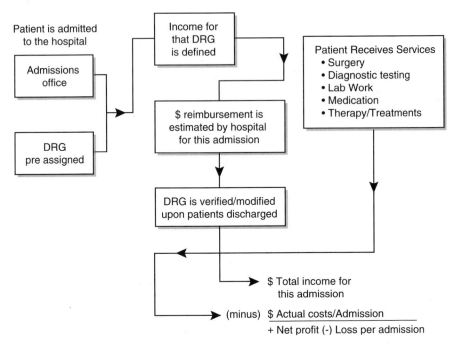

▶ **FIGURE 2–3** The prospective payment system had a significant effect on hospital administrators' desire to reduce average length of patient stay and the number of tests performed. This was because hospitals were no longer reimbursed on the basis of volume and total expenses generated by the provider.

Figure 2-3 shows a schematic of the prospective reimbursement payment system. Such a system is likely to lead to substantial pressure to reduce operating costs. As with many other industries, cutting operating costs often means cutting jobs, which can have a significant impact on our overall economy. Such cost and job cutting is occurring in health care already.

WHAT DRIVES THE SYSTEM, AND WHO IS IN THE DRIVER'S SEAT?

The health care industry pulls and pushes billions of dollars through the U.S. economy every year; however, unlike many other industries, these funds are most often not spent on elective commodities. It is a very unusual patient who is excited by the possibility of going to the hospital to receive medical services, in contrast to a consumer on his or her way to pick up a new car or dress or to make a settlement on a new boat. Clearly, the demand for health care services in most people's minds is not optional. Any system that proposes to reduce access also potentially poses a threat to our personal well-being.

The picture becomes more perplexing when we realize who is driving the system and that in most cases the consumer is totally dependent on another person for medical advice. When we realize that the adviser is actually the provider who profits from providing such services, some of the fundamental, inherent problems we have had in controlling health care costs begin to make sense. Most physicians and hospital administrators certainly have functioned with their patients' best interests in mind, but at least the potential for over-utilization of services has been omnipresent. Until recently, the entire industry was driven by the physician. It has been estimated that approximately 80% of hospital expenses is generated by the physician's pen. The physician functioned as the principal driver through the referrals he or she generated for diagnostic and treatment services. Other referrals to specialists also contributed significantly to increased health care costs. This picture is further complicated by a situation in which the provider is the most qualified person to recommend philosophical and operational guidelines to government agencies and law makers establishing guidelines for new legislation. It is little wonder that the problem of providing optimal services at the lowest cost possible has become so difficult to solve.

In addition, the author's own experiences are not unlike those of millions of others in being a parent or having parents who expect if not demand the very best treatment for these family members, giving little regard for cost of services. This expectation represents another aspect complicating the placement of controls on services. Health care reform is always more palatable when it limits access to those who are not family members; when a loved one needs medical care, limitations on access to services are not welcome in any form. In yet another variation on this, one can often hear a patient express relief that the physician he or she is seeing is extremely "thorough" as the physician "ordered everything in the book." Patients often state with pride and confidence that their test or treatment was performed with the "latest technology." The need to maintain one's personal well-being and security coupled with the referring power of the physician have clearly been significant drivers of the utilization of health care services and the associated rising costs.

COMPETITION AMONG PROVIDERS AND DEMAND FOR SERVICES

For the most part, other industries rely on open competition to regulate price, efficiency of service, availability of product, and quality. With the health care industry, products appear in the form of answers to medical questions and services provided. In addition, patients have no way of evaluating the actual appropriateness of referrals and services they receive. In fact, until recently, patients often felt a strong sense of disloyalty to their physician or hospital by even questioning these matters. In other industries working in an open market, the number of suppliers or manufacturers of a given product eventually reaches a point of equilibrium with demand, where the entry of additional providers is discouraged by dwindling profitability. At this point, business people may select another line of products to manufacture. The same is true with regard to establishing prices for their product or service. At some point equilibrium occurs, and additional increases in cost can actually reduce demand for the item.

With the health care industry, none of these check-and-balance mechanisms are in place because the decision to use services is driven by consultation with the physician and is further motivated by a strong desire to maintain one's health. The answers to the medical questions often become options for the patient to choose from. In addition, patients may select one form of surgery over another, or no surgery at all. Having a less expensive option now may led to higher costs later for the patient. One can always ratchet down the purchase of commodities, but ratcheting down the utilization NEEDED for health services is a very different matter. Health care costs are somewhat insulated from pressures of the general economy. Since most of the cost for health services is paid by insurers and not the provider/consultant or the patient, utilization is somewhat insulated from the general state of the country's economy.

However, as was pointed out earlier, the national health care bill is reaching a point relative to the GNP at which government and employers can see that health care costs should be viewed in the same context as the national debt. In fact, current projections by HCFA show that health care costs in the United States in 2005 could represent 17.9% of the country's GDP. The portion of taxes needed to cover health care will become too great a national economic burden. Employers are already beginning to demand that the increasing cost of employee health care premiums be shared by employees through lower salaries or increased co-pay insurance premiums. There is always the question of rationing other Government expenses, such as the military. However as evidenced by the legislators recently who proposed more spending for military than was requested initially, reducing funding for Medicare seems to be the preferred model.

Another important aspect of our health care system has been its monopolistic nature. The monopoly is based on the physician, who is usually affiliated with one hospital and almost requires the patient to be treated at that facility. Medical economists generally see physicians as the sole source of information needed by patients. These factors minimize patient choice, or at least willingness to request alternatives. This in turn worked to minimize competition among hospitals. As a result, there has been very little opportunity for patients to compare hospital costs.

SUPPLY OF AND DEMAND FOR HEALTH CARE SERVICES

In most industries, the conventional market pressures of supply and demand work to move price up as supplies become less available. This concept has a stabilizing effect on our general economy. In the health care system, however, supply and demand had little effect. Traditionally, patients would willingly follow their physicians' advice and demand services because services are required and the patient rarely paid the whole bill. Facilities that provided diagnostic and treatment services rarely limited supply (services) because they almost always received prevailing reimbursement rates. As long as governments can tax the population to cover Medicare and Medicaid expenses and employers can cover their employees' insurance premiums, the patient and provider remain relatively protected from conventional market forces. Health care benefits provided by employers are generally the last item to be cut from employees' benefit packages. Only the deepest recessions the country has experienced have affected the health care industry. Table 2-7A, B shows personal expenditures relative to health care.

Deciding how to deliver effective and appropriate health care services at an affordable price could become one of the country's greatest moral dilemmas. This decision will involve such difficult questions as the following:

- At what point is it appropriate to decide not to provide a service?
- Should this decision be based on patient age? For example, should the number of services an insurance group or the government covers be reduced as a patient's age advances?
- Should children receive fewer services than breadwinners?
- How do we know when the line between excessive and insufficient provision of services is crossed?

- What are the indicators of a good health care delivery system, and who should define these indicators?

Clearly, these point to complex elements and one hopes that they will never require categorical answers. However, they do point out the undeniable fact that someone must eventually pay for all health care services and that the resources available to make such payments are limited.

OTHER FACTORS THAT AFFECT DEMAND FOR SERVICES

Health care economists consider the concept of elasticity when describing demand for services. Elasticity is how sensitive a given factor is to an outside influence. If cost, for example, causes a change (increase or decrease) in the demand for a service, then we say that demand for that service has some elasticity with respect to cost (Fig. 2-4). In the case of health care, demand is expressed by the willingness of a patient to seek a medical service. Traditionally, in general industry, demand is very much related to cost. As cost goes down, interest in a product or service increases. Until recently, changes in the price of a diagnostic exam, for example, did not influence whether a patient would seek out that service. Most economists consider demand elasticity in the health care industry to be generally low. There are, however, some factors that under certain circumstances do affect demand for health care services. In fact, we began this chapter by describing some of the basic elements that pushed the rate of demand for health care in this country. However, there were relatively few factors that were in place to pull demand down.

Other out of pocket cost factors have been shown to influence demand for services within the third-party fee-for-service reimbursement system. (Fee for service in this context means that providers are paid on the basis for specific episodes or services rendered to the patient.) One of these factors is the amount of co-pay the patient will have to pay to cover what the insurance will not. Co-pay comes in a variety of forms, including paying costs entirely out of pocket or by paying costs until the deductible threshold written into a policy is reached. Other co-pay plans include the payment of additional premiums to the insurance company. Studies have shown that as the amount of co-pay increases, demand for services decreases.

A second factor that influences demand for health care services is availability. As the convenience and or availability of services to a patient increases, service utilization will tend to increase. As we will see later, availability of health care services is not totally within the control of providers; federal and state governments apply restrictions to the growth of inpatient facilities, which can come in the form of either adding a significant number of beds or building a whole new facility. Growth of outpatient services, however, is almost entirely without restraint.

Still more factors affect demand for health services. Studies of large population samples have shown that people having higher education tend to seek out medical services at a higher rate that do people having less formal education. Females have an overall higher rate of utilization of medical services than do males. Race also influences demand for medical services: Blacks tend to have a lower rate of utilization of health care services than do whites. Personal income appears not to be a significant factor affecting demand because many people of all income levels have jobs that provide health care benefits offering sufficient protection for them and their families. Clearly one group's rate of employment may result in different demands.

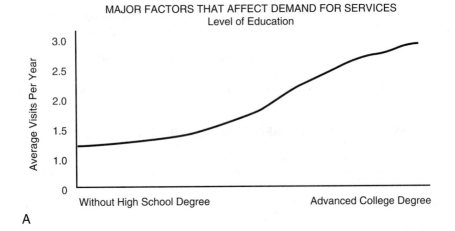

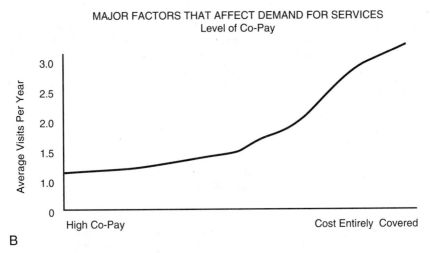

▶ **FIGURE 2–4** Shows demand curves and the concept of elasticity of demand with respect to various factors such as level of the patient's formal education and insurance coverage. In this illustration, we can see that these two factors do have an impact on the frequency with which medical services are requested.

SUBSTITUTION OF HEALTH CARE SERVICES

In the past, neither patients nor providers have been open to the idea of alternatives to traditional provision of medical services. However, more and more alternatives are emerging. A few examples can describe the idea of substitution of health care services. Over the past several years, the increased role played by specially trained nonphysicians, such as midwives, has signalled the public's acceptance of the idea of receiving critical services and care that were once squarely in the physician's domain. Another form of substitution is occurring in hospitals. Services that were once provided at significant expense over three- and four-day periods are now provided during short-stay, eight-hour admissions (Fig. 2-5). In other cases, services that were once provided during one-day admissions are now being performed on an outpatient basis. In many hospitals, surgical procedures performed on an outpatient basis are exceeding 50% of all surgical procedures performed. In 1980 approximately 16% of all surgical cases were outpatient, which rose to 55% in 1993. Cost reductions are significant: A three-day surgery admission could generate hospital costs of approximately $10,000 while a one-day, short-stay surgery admission may cost $3,500. Increased efforts to perform more procedures on a short-stay basis continue. Figure 2-6 shows average cost per discharge across the country in 1992. Figure 2-7 shows cost per inpatient day.

In the future, nurse practitioners will be used more frequently to diagnose and treat certain conditions without immediate direction from physicians. The concept and role of nurse

Community Hospitals Inpatient Days versus Outpatient Visits
1982–92

▶ **FIGURE 2−5** Much of the country began to see a trend in favor of outpatient services in the mid-1980s. This trend had a significant impact on the overall cost of medical care. In many institutions, 55% of all surgical procedures are now performed on an outpatient basis.

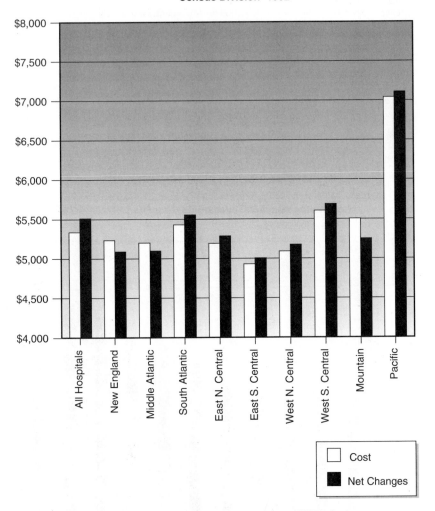

Census Division–1992

▶ **FIGURE 2–6** Shows average costs for discharge. (Courtesy of VHA, Inc.)

practitioners has been hotly debated. However, under the pressure of health care reform, there appears to be little doubt that, after graduating from special training programs, nurses will soon gain access to credentials that allow them to provide first-line care to patients. The evolution of physician's assistants is another example of substitution.

Thus, SUBSTITUTION of health care services is an evolving concept that will be given much greater emphasis by the efforts to broaden access to health care and to lower costs. Considering that in 1995 there were some 38 million people who have no access to health care that they can afford, it appears that there is enough "business" for all providers. As services are redistributed and substitutions are made, health care costs may be reined in.

Data Comparison Reporting System

Cost per Adjusted Patient Day
Second Quarter 1994

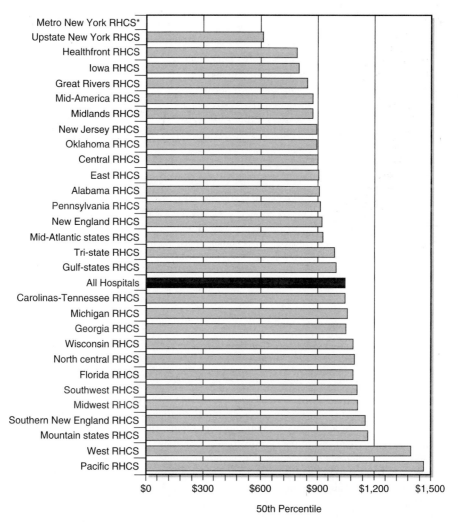

50th Percentile

▶ **FIGURE 2-7** Shows cost per adjusted patient days at various hospitals in the United States. (Source: VHA, Inc., Data Comparison Reporting System.)

MEASURING PRODUCTIVITY IN HEALTH CARE

Measuring productivity in most industries is relatively straightforward: fairly objective standards can be used as benchmarks. The health care industry, however, has proven to be a bit of an enigma in this regard. Productivity can be expressed as the relationship between utilization of resources and results over time. In the past, productivity was viewed as an il-

---

Fundamental Performance Indicators Used Regularly by Hospital Administrations

- Average length of stay
- Total patient days per year
- FTEs per staffed bed
- FTEs to outpatient tests/procedures performed
- Average cost of tests ordered per admission
- Distribution of payers
  Medicare
  Indemnity insurance companies (i.e., traditional Blue Cross, commercial payers [Prudential, Aetna & others])
  No pay
  Managed care
  Others
- Ratio of outpatient & inpatient activity by department (e.g., radiology, surgery, laboratory, other clinical services)

▶ **FIGURE 2-8** Basic operations elements hospitals often monitor to measure efficiency and to control financial standing. The ease and degree to which calculations such as these can be made routinely are dependent on the flexibility of the hospital's computer system, the skill of the people who have access to the hospital's data base, and how the information in the data base is configured.

lusive, if not inappropriate, indicator of efficiency or effectiveness of health care service. To some degree, this might have been because of the perceived sanctity of the administration of care to the sick and needy with roots going back to the almshouses.

However, questions concerning productivity in health care are certainly worthy of consideration today. How can productivity be measured? Who should set the measuring criteria? When considering productivity in the broadest sense, if we assume the elements of quality and time to be constants, the fewer resources needed to achieve the best results, the more efficient the operation. Conversely, a comparatively inefficient operation is one in which more resources are used to achieve similar or lesser results. The health care industry is generally viewed as being one of the most inefficient industries in the United States and in the world. However, this notwithstanding, in regards to the range, quality, and availability of services, our system of health care is unparalleled and the most envied in the world by those who use it. Figure 2-8 shows performance indicators regularly used by hospital administrators.

Although regimented operating standards of efficiency have been studied and published, the health care industry in the United States is moving toward a new understanding of efficiency as we build more defined models for outcome assessment. New outcome assessment criteria are being developed at many different levels throughout the country. Today, many if not most of our hospitals either have programs in place or are fast developing programs that track specific services to patients in a fashion that could only be imagined 10 years ago. Private physicians in these hospitals are continually monitored to track the number of admissions they generate and at what level of severity and for how wide a spectrum of diseases they admit patients. Once a patient is admitted, statistics on all tests, procedures, medications, treatment plans, and so forth are gathered and critically evaluated to establish their appropriateness. If these statistics show that a particular physician orders more tests than the norm, that physician is informed of this fact and asked to re-evaluate his or her protocols and practices. Refer to Figure 3-7. Outcome assessment and benchmarking are also applied to indicators of effectiveness such as the number of readmissions to a hospital and frequency of second surgical procedures for the same problem as well as to those most traditional indicators, mortality and morbidity. Such analysis can reveal much about quality of service and economic efficiency.

Vital standards that contribute to establishing overall standards are benchmark for operational efficiencies by hospital administrators. Cost comparisons are being conducted continuously among hospitals that have been networked into one system. Hospitals are also continuously comparing themselves to evolving published standards (Fig. 2-8). Overall, indicators such as the number of patient days per year and the ratio of inpatient to outpatient admissions show a declining ratio of expenses to services provided and are monitored enthusiastically.

THE COMPLEXITIES AND DANGERS INVOLVED IN CHANGING THE SYSTEM

History shows that the relationships between resources needed and results required improve under the pressure of open competition. With an industry as large and with so many complex elements driving it as the health care industry, there is no doubt that government will always be intimately involved in regulation and in funding and may take on a more controlling role than at present. Woven through all the considerations and efforts tied to health care reform lies perhaps the most central question: how to identify that elusive point of equilibrium between quality, availability or access to services, and cost. Unfortunately, government programs have not distinguished themselves as benchmarks of efficiency in either identifying or establishing those levels. To date, the movement of health care reform that has emerged from the rapid growth of managed care organizations and the speed with which we are approaching capitated contracts, defacto reform will have occurred on its own in the vacuum created by endless debates among representatives in Washington. It seems that the only questions left to government will be how to include the underserved population in this new, reformed system and how the additional associated cost will be funded.

We might consider the analogy of a balloon that has been filled with air. The air inside represents the net or hypothetical "real" demand for health care services, a kind of inherent pressure. The expanding wall of the balloon represents the strain of cost containment, a kind of backlash pressure. If pressure is applied externally to push "real" cost back and to reduce the expansion at any point of the balloon, the pressure within (demand for service) is displaced to another area of the balloon wall (Fig. 2-9). Moving or manipulating the internal demand and the external containment only redistributes the pressure points. Savings gained in one area may result in larger expenses later.

Clearly, we must be very careful when defining systems designed to decrease this demand. This job becomes particularly difficult when we consider that health care reform could involve extending access to at least an additional 38 million people. The problem is also complex because there are so many elements within the health care industry that clear causes and effects are difficult to foresee on a long term basis. There are secondary elements to the problem that may not be apparent initially but that may surface many years later. For example, if access to services is broadened to include those not covered today but costs are not increased substantially, fewer pieces of equipment per capita may be available and long delays in the scheduling of procedures may result. As more—and older—people are insured to cover hospitalization at the same time controls on costs tighten, elective or marginally elective admissions will likely be delayed. As the government makes fewer dollars avail-

FACTORS THAT AFFECT DEMAND FOR MEDICAL SERVICES

- Skill/Philosophy of Medical Advisors
  - Advice Sought From Physician Specialist
  - Advice Sought From Physician in Family Practice
- Degree of Co-Pay
  (Ranges Between Services Being Provided)
  - Totally Insured
  - Partially Insured
  - Not Insured At All
- Availability of Services Needed
  - Location of Facility
  - Long Scheduling Delays
  - Convenience/Amenities Offered by Facility
- Age of Population
- Perceived Risk of Not Seeking Care
- Personal Life Style
  - Education
  - Income Level
- Facility/Management Profile
  - Initiatives Taken to Reduce Utilization/Expenses of Services
  - Operational Efficiencies
  - Degree/Level of Reimbursement

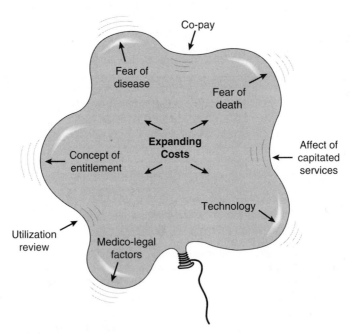

▶ **FIGURE 2-9** Shows some of the major factors that affect demand for services. As these factors expand or retreat, demand for health care often change. These factors have a variety of effects on cost and demand for services and sometimes constitute complex relationships.

able to universities to fund medical research, fewer advances may result. The preface of this book clearly defines that the engineers of change in health are actually our congressmen and senators, whose own motives may obscure a clear view to the second and third level of outcome for patients who are not in a position to argue for themselves.

The aggregate impact of changes aimed to effect health care system reform may be devastating to people who do not receive the *right* mix of insurance coverage. As health care reform proceeds, reductions in demand for services, increased monitoring for appropriateness of services rendered, substitutions, and a multitude of other changes must be implemented in correct order and each to its proper degree because of the complexity of the health care industry and the serious impact miscalculations would have on those who depend on services. Certainly, this period of transition is at the very least interesting because it is forcing each of us to evaluate some of our most personal values. The process of defining measurements and values in such a way as to maintain our personal well-being will continue for many more years.

OTHER PRODUCTIVITY CONSIDERATIONS

It is difficult to establish objective productivity calculations for the health care industry. This does not mean that it is not possible to do so, but it does mean that additional care should be taken to account for a wide variety of variables. For example, each disease has its own intensity rate among various age groups and between the sexes. Not all patients recover at the same rate despite consistent delivery of care (Table 2-8). Patient mortality and morbidity have been used widely to measure effectiveness of care; yet effectiveness of care may not necessarily provide clear answers to questions regarding productivity and efficiency. For example, a higher than average morbidity or mortality rate at one hospital could mean that sufficient quality of care is being rendered but that the population of patients seen at the facility is more prone to complications.

▶ TABLE 2–8
TRENDS IN DEATH RATES

DISEASE GROUPS	1970	1990
Heart	258.6	152
Cerebrovascular	66.3	27.7
Malignancies	129.9	135
Chronic obstructive	[1980]	
pulmonary disease	15.9	8.6
Pneumonia & Influenza	22.1	14

NOTE: Death rates above shown per 100,000 cases
(Source: U.S. National Center for Health Statistics.)

Indicates that over the last 20 years, death rates for these select diseases have shown improvement. These rates, however, are not stellar when compared to those of other well-developed countries that have less costly health care systems. The United States's mortality and morbidity rates, especially for newborns, do not compare favorably with other countries'. They have, however, shown improvement since 1994.

► TABLE 2-9
LIFE EXPECTANCY AND INFANT MORTALITY RATES

| | YEARS OF LIFE EXPECTANCY | | INFANT MORTALITY: |
COUNTRY	1986	1991	% IMPROVEMENT BETWEEN 1986 AND 1991
Canada	73.1	74.4	3.4%
England	72.6	73.5	6.8%
Germany	69.5	69.3	3.2%
Japan	75.5	76.4	1.4%
United States	71	72	1.6%

Source: National Center for Health Statistics, *Public Health Services.*

A brief comparison of life expectancies and infant mortality rates of the United States and other industrialized countries.

Impact studies have been used to evaluate the cause-and-effect relationships of various treatment plans. For example, Hadley's impact studies demonstrated that, for a sample group of 200,000 people, an increase of 1% in medical expenditures resulted in a 0.16% reduction in mortality. One may question the sensitivity of these parameters to each other, but not their cause and effect. As more information like this is evaluated, we should work to build protocols that will lead to more appropriate or more effective utilization of resources. Health economists are continually searching for optimal combinations of various elements within the health care system in order to reach the point of equilibrium between acceptable access to service, outcome, and cost.

For example, somewhere in these combinations might lie answers to such questions of cost effectiveness as how much money to spend for new technology to treat cancer versus how much money should be spent on population education and prevention efforts. There may be a more appropriate balance that has not been achieved. Consider, for instance, how the money spent for increased education of the public about the dangers of cigarette smoking and exposure to carcinogens in our everyday life has affected morbidity and mortality rates. Educational programs concerning diet may reduce the incidence rates of certain diseases at a cost much lower than that for the procedures, personnel, and equipment needed to treat these diseases. A certain amount of money spent on educational programs about early detection of breast and colon cancer may result in a more dramatic reduction of cancer mortality rates than will more money spent on developing new treatment programs or equipment. A number of investigations have shown that Medicare expenditures can affect mortality. For example, it has been demonstrated that a 1% increase in spending will result in a 0.2% to 0.4% reduction in mortality among whites and a 0.5% to 1.0% reduction among blacks. But these studies are not enough. A universal set of criteria that will more effectively measure health status and, ultimately, productivity and outcome of services has yet to be fully defined. Table 2-9 summarizes life expectancy and infant mortality statistics in the United States and other industrialized countries.

CONSUMERISM IN THE HEALTH CARE INDUSTRY

No discussion of the health care delivery system would be complete without addressing consumerism. Many economists argue that the health care industry presently lacks sufficiently developed consumerism. First, the average patient has little knowledge or expertise concerning what constitutes quality of service and how it should be measured. Second, patients and providers have rarely balanced cost of service provided against outcome. Finally, long-standing patient loyalty to personal physicians as trusted medical advisers and even personal confidants has blunted patient scrutiny of medical costs and services.

THE BASIS OF POOR CONSUMERISM

A study performed by Grossman in 1972 showed that what people seek as the result of receiving health care services is not the act of receiving such services itself but rather the state of healthfulness. This finding may help to explain why people have traditionally been relatively uninterested in the specific service received—it is only a means to the desired end and therefore takes on only passing significance. Another point this study made is that patients place high value on the personal input required of them as they pursue that state of healthfulness. Input in this context is any effort a patient must invest to receive service, which may include driving long distances to unfamiliar locations or walking through strange, sprawling health care facilities. This effort sometimes demands fortitude, particularly of elderly and disabled patients. Such input may also involve time and miscellaneous expenses for travel, parking, and meals. In other words, patients are very mindful of the time, inconvenience, and personal expense they incur when seeking health care services. As the level of patient input required increases, the less interest patients will show in seeking out services.

A third concept that this study exposed is that health care is not an episodic occurrence; it is instead an ongoing maintenance program. In a business sense, health care should be compared to a long-term capital reinvestment program rather than to a one-time purchase. It is appropriate to consider that, in addition to increasing piece of mind, good health care offers such benefits as allowing us to enjoy leisure time, to generate income, and to enjoy the company of family and friends to the fullest. Thus, as patients, each of us has become an investor in a state of healthfulness for ourselves and for the members of our families. This can lead us to an increased appreciation of preventive care such as routine checkups, better diets, stress-reduction measures, and worthwhile exercise programs. A good state of healthfulness is an economic investment for the country as well because it allows us to work and earn income, which generates taxes and allows us to purchase goods and services.

THE PHYSICIAN-PATIENT RELATIONSHIP

The relationship between the physician and the patient in the United States is interesting and unique among industrialized countries. Patients, even in today's enlightened age, still tend to view their physicians as confidants and trusted medical consultants. Patients seek advice and care that will determine their state of healthfulness. In addition, this advice concerns a subject matter that is usually quite beyond the patient's understanding. Patients' ability to seek information sufficient to allow them to critique physicians' recommendations is thus very limited.

This model in which the physician acts as sole provider of critical health information is, however, breaking down in the 1990s. Patient's rights to seek advice and to receive other forms of medical care are becoming clearer, and what has been described as an aloof or marginally sympathetic attitude among physicians is being challenged more aggressively each year. More and more patients are expecting higher levels of personal attention from their physicians (as compared to the days of rapidly emerging technology and specialization), and physicians are becoming more aware of emerging patient expectations. Patients are expressing this expectation by seeking second opinions and by switching physicians when they are dissatisfied. As HMOs and capitated reimbursement contracts become more and more prevalent, the physician's role as an independent adviser is expected to diminish significantly. This is because physicians working within HMO guidelines are expected to follow established treatment plans and regimens that have been developed over time by an HMO's medical panel rather than by the individual physician.

CONSUMERISM CONCERNING INSTITUTIONS

Health care institutions are also reacting to new patient expectations. Hospital administrators, and members of their boards of trustees, are placing a much stronger emphasis on making their services more convenient, more pleasant, and less costly. Hospitals are now enthusiastically utilizing patient survey results, advertising their services, and increasing the level of expertise of their medical staffs and other employees. Hospital quality management departments are conducting focused studies by calling groups of patients back to the hospital to discuss the pros and cons of the services they have received. Figure 2-10 is an example of a survey that many hospitals use to evaluate their services. Patients are also becoming more aware of their "Bill of Rights," which in most hospitals is given to patients during the admission process (Fig. 2-11).

ADVERTISING, THE NEW REVOLUTION

Until recently, to advertise medical services was considered at least tacky if not an outright display that the advertiser was lacking in ethics. Is advertising health care services appropriate? If so, what is the optimal level of advertising? The pharmaceutical industry has advertised over-the-counter medications openly for many years. How can the larger health services industry advertise its services, which are complex, while staying within ethical bounds?

An advertising campaign may deal with the type of product that is being offered, its costs, availability, quality, and price. These characteristics can be more easily identified and quantified for common commodities than for a service that has many intangible aspects. Health care services must be advertised in a very different way. For example, it has been shown that patients who respond to surveys regarding hospital services they have received less often address aspects of care that involve quality of diagnosis, quality or capability of equipment, or even quality of treatment. They most often address aspects that involve personal comfort, personal convenience, and mannerisms of staff. They cannot measure the former items because they don't have the necessary expertise. They do understand the latter aspects of care, and this is often where most of their complaints are aimed. Thus, an advertising campaign may be more effective if it addresses the latter aspects and lets the patient assume that the former aspects are fine. The designer of a health care service advertising campaign should therefore know the answers to the following questions:

1. Who are the customers or target group?
2. Are they the correct target group for the service being provided?
3. How large is the customer base?
4. What are the customers' needs?
5. What services will satisfy those needs?

Overall Hospital Questions
Patient's Name
Room Number
Date of Admission
Age   Sex
Telephone Number

Admission
• Efficiency of admission process
• Courtesy of personnel
• Did you have excessive delays?
Comments: _____

_____

Your Stay on the Nursing Floor
• Appearance of your room
• Level of comfort you had while in the room
• Cleanliness of the room
• General appearance of the room
• Degree of privacy provided
• TV, phone, lighting, comfort of bed
• Courtesy of those who cleaned your room
Comments: _____

_____

Food
• Did you understand your diet?
• Quality and taste of food your were served
• Did you receive the selections you requested?

Nursing Staff
• Nursing and friendliness of nurses
• Did they respond promptly when needed?
• Did nurses take your concerns seriously?
• Were you kept informed about up-coming events?
• How do you assess the skill and knowledge of the nurses?
Comments: _____

_____

Tests and Procedures
• Courtesy of staff who performed your tests
• Length of time you waited before your tests
• Length of time you waited after your tests to return to your room

• How do you assess the skill and knowledge of the technologists?
• Did the technologists adequately explain the test to you?
• Were your concerns taken seriously?
Comments: _____

_____

Other
• Helpfulness of volunteers
• Helpfulness of staff in general
• Would you recommend this hospital?
• Degree to which you feel nurses and other departments coordinated your tests during your stay
Comments: _____

_____

Services Provided to Visitors
• Courtesy of people at the information desk
• General accommodations and help given to visitors
• Was family kept adequately informed and involved?
Comments: _____

_____

Your Physician
• Did you have sufficient time with your doctor?
• Was he/she available when needed?
• Did he/she provide the information that you needed?
• Courtesy of other physicians who attended to you
Comments: _____

_____

Discharge Process
• Did you have adequate notice of your discharge?
• Efficiency of the discharge process
• Was your discharge coordinated properly?
• Were you provided with the information you needed for caring for yourself before discharge?
Comments: _____

_____

▶ **FIGURE 2–10** Shows a typical inpatient satisfaction survey.

Patient Bill of Rights

The General Hospital is committed to excellence in patient service. Our physicians and personnel recognize that effective communication with the patient and his/her family is an important part of any treatment plan as is cooperation by the patient and his/her family.

As a patient, you have the right to:

1. Reasonable and respectful care by competent personnel;
2. Access to an interpreter if necessary;
3. Privacy and confidentiality of care;
4. Confidentiality regarding medical records and communications;
5. Be informed by your physician of all diagnoses, treatment and prognoses, in understandable terms;
6. Care without unnecessary delay and with the least physical discomfort possible;
7. The names of all physicians and other caregivers involved with your treatment;
8. Refuse any drugs, treatments or procedures and participation in clinical research programs;
9. Consult with another physician;
10. Be transferred to another facility;
11. Assistance in planning for your care after your release;
12. An explanation of your bill and financial counseling;
13. Quality medical care monitored by the hospital's Quality Assessment and Improvement Program;
14. Access the information in your medical records;
15. Care without discrimination based on race, color, religion, sex, sexual preference, national origin or source of payment;
16. Access to an individual or agency authorized to act on your behalf;
17. Be informed of your rights;
18. Express dissatisfaction with the care or services you received without fear of repercussions;
19. Expedient review and resolution of any complaint.

As a patient, parent or legal guardian, you play an active role in the treatment your child receives. We ask that you:

1. Provide a complete medical history;
2. Cooperate with hospital personnel and ask questions if you do not understand directions;
3. Respect the rights of other patients;
4. Provide the necessary insurance information;
5. Be responsible for your personal property;
6. Help in your or your child's care by following all instructions;

▶ **FIGURE 2−11** Identifies elements of a patient's rights that all patients and employees should understand.

> **The relationship between you and your physician is essential to your recovery. Therefore, both the patient and the physician have the right to terminate the relationship at any time. Here are some possible reasons terminating the relationship might be considered:**
> 1. Incompatibility of personalities;
> 2. The patient's illness is beyond the physician's expertise;
> 3. Excessive consultation with other physicians without the knowledge and consent of the primary physician;
> 4. Repeated failure to follow physician's advice and treatment.

▶ **FIGURE 2–11** *Continued*

6. Who and where is the competition?

7. How can one's service be differentiated from the competition's?

8. Does the mission of the service and our objectives match the customers' needs? (Are we providing a service that we should not be involved in?)

Hospitals first began advertising their services in the mid-1960s by creating development departments. These departments were closely linked to hospital administrations. Their mission was and still is to promote their facilities' services to the public. In addition, they attempt to generate good will in the community toward the hospital and to attract donations. Development departments grew rapidly in popularity and increased in numbers in the mid-1980s by 74 percent. Although this form of advertising was more subtle than that which we see today, it was nevertheless effective, and it resulted in getting information to the general public and to the business community.

Initially, development departments and hospitals were not very interested in advertising (in the conventional sense) their services. The American Hospital Association (AHA) raised ethical questions to the extent that pressure was applied to reduce advertising by member hospitals. This was, however, challenged, and the federal courts ruled that efforts by an organization, in this case the AHA, to reduce or limit advertising amounted to restraint of trade and was therefore against the law. Despite this ruling, questions are still raised regarding the possible violation of patients' trust in an institution (Fig. 2-12). However, a survey conducted by the AMA in 1984 indicated that 62 percent of those surveyed felt that advertising increased their ability to choose services.

Perhaps the principal advantage advertising offers a patient is that information associated with identifying choices. It may also increase patient interest in seeking better and less expensive services. Because health care is not necessarily a wanted service, as are most commodities, health care advertising has a slightly different tone and purpose. It is certain that health care advertising has now gained acceptance, and over the next several years, it may prove a significant source of public information and education. Now that advertising is making information more available, the public should take its share of responsibility and become more knowledgeable about the options it has when choosing the who, what, where, and why aspects of the health care services it receives.

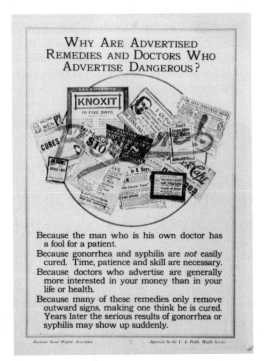

WHY ARE ADVERTISED
REMEDIES AND DOCTORS WHO
ADVERTISE DANGEROUS?

Because the man who is his own doctor has a fool for a patient.
Because gonorrhea and syphilis are *not* easily cured. Time, patience and skill are necessary.
Because doctors who advertise are generally more interested in your money than in your life or health.
Because many of these remedies only remove outward signs, making one think he is cured. Years later the serious results of gonorrhea or syphilis may show up suddenly.

▶ **FIGURE 2−12** Indicates the level of acceptability that advertising health care services had in the past. (Source: National Library of Medicine.)

BUILDING AN EFFECTIVE SERVICE

There are those who believe that the best advertisement is the provision of a high-quality, cost-effective service—which leaves the responsibility for the success of an advertising campaign resting squarely on operations managers. The reality is that neither the service nor the advertising campaign can be used solely to support the other. Both the advertising effort and the service must satisfy the customer. In effect, a blueprint for service must be developed and implemented. Developing a blueprint for each given service requires a substantial investment of time and research.

Fundamental Steps to Developing a Blueprint for Service

1. Identify the service you provide.
2. Identify your customer(s).
3. Identify the objectives of an optimal service.
4. Identify the criteria that will be used to measure success in meeting objectives.
5. Develop an operations plan for attaining these objectives.
6. Develop a method for monitoring continued compliance.

The key to success throughout this process is not to over- or underestimate the complexity of the problem as we will see in Chapter Six.

Because the customer is the most important element of this process, the primary criteria that count are those the customer (patient, physician, family, another department, etc.) defines for the health care worker. Thus, the quality and effectiveness of service will eventually be measured by the criteria the customer perceives to be important. These discussions are used to get firsthand impressions of and insights on what worked for the patients and what did not. These data are then summarized and carried back to the department or service to work into its operations plan. In this sense, the customer can become a codesigner of future services.

Ultimately, the following five elements must be built into the blueprint:

- Superior appearance, comfort, and convenience of the facility
- Reliability of the service
- Responsiveness to the customer's needs
- Competence of personnel
- Courtesy of personnel
- Timeliness of the services provided

STUDY QUESTIONS

1. Write a brief advertisement for a hospital you know, and develop a slogan that best carries the message you want the public to receive about the service(s) your hospital provides.

2. List five fundamental patient rights that you think every patient should know about and exercise. Compare these to a copy of the Bill of Rights published by a local hospital, and discuss how patients and hospital personnel should be made aware of this important document.

3. Explain consumerism as it relates to health care delivery and what you think patients could do to further this movement. Also discuss changes that can be made in health care delivery that could improve the quality of information and its availability to patients. To what degree should consumerism be advanced by a hospital?

4. Describe alternatives for spending health care money, aside from new technology and techniques for treating and diagnosing disease, that would benefit patients. What measures do you think should be taken to increase application of these alternatives?

5. Briefly define a method for evaluating the effectiveness of a specific service, such as radiology, for its patients within a hospital. What specific criteria would you use to measure effectiveness and quality of service?

6. What is substitution as it relates to health care delivery? Give two examples. Make some judgment concerning the appropriateness of application of substitution, and consider how substitution might evolve over the next five years.

Summary of Expenditures for Research in Health Care					
Past, Present, and Future Estimates					
(Expressed in Billions of Dollars)					
5.5	7.8	12.2	15.9	19.6	24.4
1980	1985	1990	1995	2000	2005

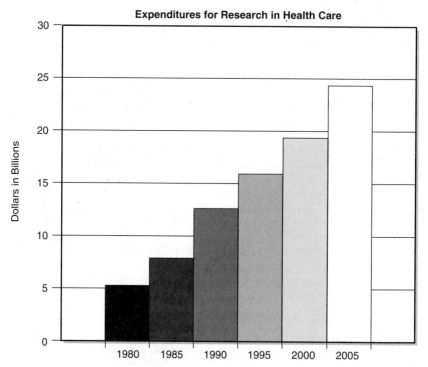

▶ **FIGURE 2–13** Research aimed at advancing medical care is largely funded by the National Institutes of Health (NIH). Such research has provided immeasurable benefit to patients directly and to nonpatients indirectly. As you can see, however, these efforts are not inexpensive. (Source: Health Care Financing Administration, Office of the Actuary, and National Health Statistics.)

Summary of Expenditures for Construction in Health Care					
Past, Present, and Future Estimates					
(Expressed in Billions of Dollars)					
6.2	8.6	12.1	14.2	16.5	20
1980	1985	1990	1995	2000	2005

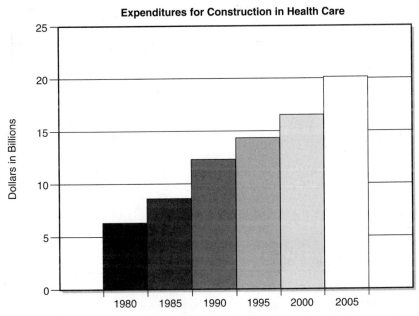

Expenditures for Construction in Health Care

▶ **FIGURE 2–14** Shows past, present, and projected expenditures associated with construction of health care facilities. (Source: Health Care Financing Administration, Office of the Actuary, and National Health Statistics.)

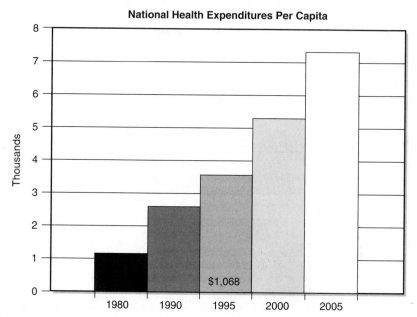

National Health Expenditures Per Capita				
$1,068	$2,686	$3,685	$5,198	$7,352
1980	1990	1995	2000	2005

▶ **FIGURE 2-15** Shows national health care expenditures per capita. (Source: Health Care Financing Administration, Office of the Actuary, and National Health Statistics.)

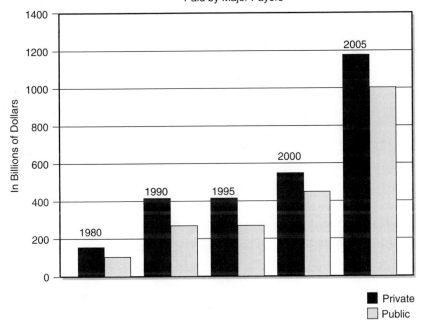

National Health Expenditures
Paid by Major Payers

▶ **FIGURE 2−16** Shows distribution of payments by major health care payers. Public payers are federal, state, and local governments. (Source: Health Care Financing Administration, Office of the Actuary.)

THREE

The Hospital as an Organized and Integrated System

OBJECTIVES FOR STUDY

After reading this chapter, the student will

▶ Understand the fundamental factors that drive political and economic decisions in hospitals.

▶ Understand the role of the board of directors in hospitals and its relationship with key administrative and medical staff personnel.

▶ Appreciate the various internal and external factors that significantly affect hospital policy and planning strategies.

▶ Understand the various types of hospital corporations and their administrative structures.

▶ Understand the fundamental organizational structure of the medical staff within a hospital.

▶ Appreciate the characteristics of community, tertiary-care, and university-based hospitals.

INTRODUCTION

As we have learned, the health care system, and hospitals in particular, had a very fragmented beginning. In the earliest stages of their development, some hospitals were nothing more than halfway houses for passersby who needed a place to stay, food, and minor medical care. They were funded by philanthropists and physicians and operated as charitable facilities. They actually provided relatively little medical care: They were staffed by non-skilled volunteers who had little access to books or printed materials that would improve their limited medical education and understanding of the most fundamental elements of the causes and effects of disease.

Other facilities emerged that took on the task of caring for the mentally impaired. For the most part, such organizations provided a way to segregate these people from the general population and to provide basic room and board. History books describe early beliefs among the general population that mental illness was a sign of a lack of divinity within the person and even represented the presence of the devil. Given these beliefs, the separation of the mentally impaired from the general public and an inhumane level of care by today's standards was inevitable. In some of these facilities, the conditions were appalling, while others provided better care and attention than a mentally impaired person would have received anywhere else.

Today, medical care has evolved into a substantial industry that generates $938.3 billion in expenses annually. The annual operating budget of a moderately sized (450-bed) hospital might be about $125 million, while a large university-based hospital might have an operating budget of approximately $300 million. Hospitals have become very complex and sophisticated in the range of services they provide as they participate in active research programs designed to meet demands for better ways to diagnose and treat diseases.

EXTERNAL INFLUENCING FACTORS

Hospitals have today become one of the most difficult organizations to manage (Fig. 3-1). In part, this is because health care is one of the most highly regulated industries in the country in addition to being one of the industries most vulnerable to the impact of community opinions. These regulations impose not only limits for payment for services, but also rigid guidelines for virtually every procedure performed within the institution. In addition to the regulatory agencies, two other important elements have a very significant effect on the administration and financial activities of a hospital. These are the medical staff and the larger community, which includes business people and patients.

The relationship between the medical staff and the hospital administration creates a mixture of demands and dependencies that can generate considerable emotion and political pressure within each of and between these two groups. On the one hand, the medical staff depends on the hospital to provide a facility that is adequately staffed and equipped because without such a facility, doctors would not be able to perform their diagnostic and treatment services. In this regard, the hospital maintains a controlling influence on when and how physicians practice medicine and even on what services they can provide. On the other hand, the hospital depends on physicians to refer patients to it. Without these referrals, the hospital could not generate income. The political balance of maintaining good will among physicians who refer patients to the facility is very difficult while significant pressure is applied by administration for physicians to reduce operating costs of the hospital.

The larger community is the second element that plays a significant role in determining how the hospital will function. Most hospitals are structured as not-for-profit corporations, a status that will be discussed in more detail later. In addition, hospitals are actually bound

---

Overview of External Influences on Decision Making

I. Community
   - Rotary & other business organizations
   - Chamber of Commerce
II. Government
   - State regulatory agencies
   - Federal regulatory agencies
   - Legislation pending, future
III. Payers
   - Pending and future HMO contracts
   - Medicare & Medicaid legislation
IV. Regulatory agencies
   - Utilization review organizations
   - HMOs
   - Joint commission
   - Peer review
V. Economic trends
   - Increasing national pressure for health care reform

▶ **FIGURE 3–1** Unlike managers in most major industries, hospital administrators are vulnerable to the influence of these external elements, must be seriously considered and woven into the hospital's short- and long-range planning strategies.

and held to function in the community's trust, and therefore must function as the custodians of the community's health care resources. This is especially true in communities where there is only one hospital to provide these services. You will see in Chapter Four, when we discuss the financial aspects of hospital management in more detail, how maintaining the community's trust plays a significant role in defining the scope of services a hospital may provide. The author has witnessed on several occasions how communities, through strong political pressure, have persuaded hospitals not to implement new programs and services. In this text, these two major factors, the medical staff and the community, will be considered external to hospital administration, despite the significant level of influence they have on its operations and decision making.

Hospital administrations are often viewed as reactionary and bureaucratic as compared to the managements of for-profit industries. However, no other industry must be so intimately concerned with such external factors as:

- Highly regulated and closely monitored activities
- Medical staff needs
- Strong community interest
- Laws that could significantly affect future financial and operations decisions as well as income
- Laws that change the payment structure significantly

These factors can impede quick decision making.

**Overview of Internal Influences
on Decision Making**

I. Board of directors
  • Budget
  • Mission statement
  • Organization culture
  • Scope & quality of services
II. Administration
  • Resource managers
  • Monitors effectiveness of services
  • Allocates resources
III. Medical staff
  • Defines need for services
  • Utilizes resources

▶ **FIGURE 3–2** Typical elements that must be considered when planning operational strategies. Sometimes the basic internal influences shown here are not completely compatible with external pressures and surprisingly energetic conflicts result.

INTERNAL INFLUENCING FACTORS

Hospital operations are driven by three major entities that must work together effectively on a day-to-day basis to provide needed patient services. These are the board of directors, the medical staff, and the hospital administration, and we will now discuss their composition and functions (Fig. 3-2). We will begin at the top of the ladder in regards to responsibility by describing the board of directors. This body may operate under titles such as board of governors or board of trustees. As in other corporations, this body is responsible for setting overall policies, direction, and strategies for the institution. It is not involved in day-to-day operating decisions per se, but its influence can be seen in almost every decision made by the administration. For instance, it is responsible for developing and approving decisions on global issues such as the hospital's strategic plan. Because they work for a not-for-profit corporation, the directors are not responsible for maximizing profits for shareholders, which is the bottom-line responsibility of their counterparts in the for-profit business world. But the board is legally held responsible by the community for all health care-related operations within the hospital. In general, this responsibility includes:

1. The quality of care given
2. The scope of services provided
3. The efficiency of services provided
4. The provision of these services at the lowest cost possible

FOR-PROFIT AND NOT-FOR-PROFIT HOSPITALS

A hospital is usually structured in one of three basic ways:

• Private for-profit
• Private not-for-profit
• Public (federal, state, county, or city government) not-for-profit

For-profit hospitals function in exactly the same corporate manner as any other for-profit business. Their principal goal is to maximize profits in order to generate favorable returns for their investors. They also work to improve their overall marketing positions to improve their financial underpinnings. Compared to not-for-profit facilities, they claim relatively little community affiliation in the philanthropic sense. For instance, as for-profit businesses, such hospitals may object to treating patients who cannot pay for medical care. Another key difference between private for-profit and not-for-profit hospitals is that for-profit hospitals must pay taxes just as other for-profit businesses must.

Not-for-profit hospitals pay no taxes on their income, although this practice is being debated in many communities. An important difference between for-profit and not-for-profit hospitals is that, because for-profit hospitals are in business to make money for their shareholders, they can use their net revenue over expenses for any purpose. In contrast, not-for-profit hospitals are in theory owned by the community, and any net revenue over expenses must be rolled back into the organization to assure availability of current and new services to the community. These surplus funds can be plowed into new construction designed to support health care services or invested for other future use by the community. Such investments help assure that equipment and facilities will be available to provide for future health care needs.

COMPOSITION OF THE BOARD

The strength of the board of directors lies in the diversity of its membership, which usually comes from a pool of highly skilled candidates. Some hospitals pay board members, but most boards are composed of volunteers. Being a member of the board of directors carries a measure of prestige. Board members have a high level of responsibility as advocates for the community's health needs, so serving on the board provides its members with an opportunity to take an active role in determining how health care services will be provided in the community. Many individuals therefore feel honored to be asked to serve; for this reason, the pool of highly skilled business people from which to draw members is usually very deep.

The diversity of its membership contributes significantly to the board's character, effectiveness, and leadership capabilities, and these in turn determine how the hospital will carry out its duties and define its mission. In the author's experience, the membership is in fact very aware of and does carry out its responsibility to the community. The board is in fact legally bound to uphold its responsibility to develop resources and provide appropriate health care for the community.

There are relatively few specific criteria that one must meet in order to be eligible for board membership. Candidates for board positions are often recruited by incumbent board members, hospital administrators, physicians, and members of the business community. In general, a candidate must

1. Be a member in good standing of the community;
2. Possess a basic interest in work as a volunteer and be committed to accepting the legal responsibilities and to putting in the necessary hours of work; and
3. And possess the leadership skills needed to make unbiased decisions for the hospital on behalf of the community interest.

Moreover, because the board also breaks into subcommittees to perform certain activities or tasks, candidates are often selected on the basis of a particular skill or set of experiences that may benefit the research, analytical, and approval stages of various decisions that the board anticipates making.

Boards of directors are typically composed of community and business leaders, physicians, attorneys, members of the clergy, and accountants. The membership is typically heavily weighted by business leaders. There are no specific training criteria for new board members, although the American Hospital Association offers well-developed programs and other information to help fledgling board members better understand their duties and responsibilities. In many cases, mentoring relationships develop and new members receive on-the-job training. Other training is provided by seminars for newly appointed board members.

RESPONSIBILITIES OF THE BOARD

The board must direct the hospital in such a way that it responsibly addresses the issues of the quality, scope, efficiency, and cost of services provided. The board is especially responsible to the community for patient safety and quality of care. A landmark legal decision came in 1965 in the case of *Darling v. Charleston Hospital,* in which, for the first time, a hospital board was held responsible for mistreatment of a patient by a physician. This case also created a precedent such that boards were to be held legally responsible for certain actions of hospital physicians and other employees. As we will see later, this precedent in effect gave boards the right and responsibility to review physician credentials and to give final approval to each physician before his or her official appointment to the medical staff. It also gave boards authority to set policy for care provided by physicians while working in their institutions.

THE MEDICAL STAFF

The medical staff also has a very diverse membership. As noted above, a physician must be approved and credentialed by the board of directors before he or she can practice medicine in a hospital or be given admitting privileges. The medical staff operates using a charter that spells out the bylaws of the medical staff organization and the staff's rights and privileges regarding the practice of medicine within the hospital. There are several different medical groups that function within the medical staff. These include surgeons, internists, general practitioners, psychiatrists, and others. The medical staff has a self-governing body, and its organization structure is shown in Figure 3-3.

In most hospitals, individual physicians and the medical staff as a whole function outside the line management structure of the hospital administration. They are answerable to the chief of staff, who in many institutions functions as an adviser to the hospital administration. Today, however, many hospitals employ a physician who works full-time as an adviser on medical issues and to resolve medical staff–administrative issues. This physician usually carries a title such as Vice President of Medical Affairs. In some hospitals, the VP MD also functions as a line manager for the chairperson of each medical department in the hospital. The various chiefs of these medical services will usually report either to the VP of Medical Affairs, who is a full-time employee of the hospital's administrative staff. This reporting relationship applies to matters and procedures that impact the hospital's realistic well-being, but does not hold for business matters and operating decisions within a group's private practice.

Thus, the medical staff has a dual function. In one function, it must fulfill its obligation to work effectively with the hospital administration and board of directors. In the other, each physician on staff must satisfy the rules of the staff's own governance as defined by its charter and bylaws (Fig. 3-4). One can see from Figure 3-4 that the medical staff structure is

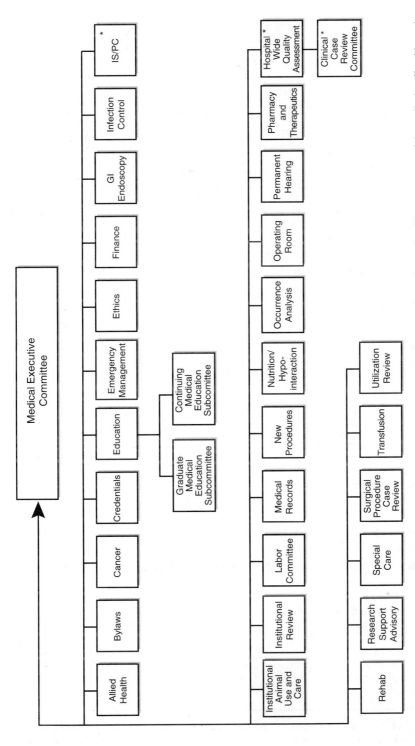

▲ **FIGURE 3-3** The structure of the medical staff at a typical hospital is much more complex than many realize. The governance of the medical staff and its various committees is mandated by hospital boards and various regulatory agencies. The time physicians must spend in committee work represents a very substantial investment in the organization.

▶ **FIGURE 3–4** Table of contents of a typical medical staff's rules of governance, which establish the need for a variety of committees. Many of these committees are required by regulatory agencies.

quite complex. One should also keep in mind that supporting and maintaining this vital entity within the hospital requires significant effort and commitment of time from many medical staff members, particularly those who hold key roles within this structure.

At university-based hospitals, the medical staff structure is slightly different. Here, the hospital is often a division of the university's medical school. Its medical program is often considerably larger and substantially more complex than those at non-university-based hospitals because of the medical school and its associated research and teaching activities. Within the configuration of a university-based medical center, we may find the medical school, the hospital, its research programs, and multiple outpatient clinics. Also, many physicians are members of the medical school faculty. They carry faculty titles such as Assistant Professor, Associate Professor, or Professor of Radiology. Each medical specialty has a department chairperson who carries the title of Professor. Not all physicians in the university setting, however, have faculty appointments. Most physicians practice within one of the services as private physicians who have met all the criteria for being members of the university's medical staff. These physicians make up various practicing groups on staff who answer to the chairpersons of their specialties, such as the chairperson of orthopedic surgery. There may, for instance, be several orthopedic groups on staff who are governed by the university through the chairperson of orthopedic surgery. The various department chairpersons in turn report to the dean of medicine, and the dean of medicine reports to the university president.

BUSINESS ASPECTS OF THE MEDICAL STAFF

As we will see in later chapters, physicians sometimes work as employees of hospitals and receive salaries for their services as employees. Under these circumstances, the hospital submits what is termed a "global" bill, which includes the technical (hospital) and professional (physician) charges. Although this practice is unusual today, there is a trend toward using salaried physicians who are fully employed by the hospital.

Although many physicians prefer to operate as private practitioners, many physicians are becoming disenchanted with private practice because nonmedical requirements are becoming a larger and larger part of their activities. More demanding legislation, hospital procedural rules, and payer requirements impose a matrix of business-related paperwork that takes a significant amount of time away from the practice of medicine. In addition, because of changing reimbursement structures, many practices are having serious financial difficulties. The combination of these factors creates an environment in which hospitals have opportunities to buy practices as one might purchase a business. When this occurs, the hospital manages the practice and handles all the associated paperwork, which frees the physicians of these nuisances. The hospital pays the physicians salaries. As we will see later, under certain reimbursement models, it is important not only to keep referrals, but also to have a correct mix of types of admissions. Many hospitals today are operating at between 40% and 70% of their total bed capacity. With this in mind, a hospital may decide to buy a particular practice to help assure that the number or mix of admissions to the institution is properly maintained in order to reinforce the institution's financial viability. In many instances a hospital will carefully identify a group practice or single physician to buy out with this balanced case mix in mind.

HOSPITAL ADMINISTRATION

We sometimes speak of an administrative triad within a hospital (Fig. 3-5). The triad is composed of the board of directors, the medical staff, and the hospital administration. As

Fundamental Complexity of Hospital Operations
Hospital Triad

Overall Responsibilities

Board of Directors

- Responsible for providing quality of medical services to the community

- Responsible for defining overall strategic planning and direction for the hospital

- Responsible for providing an appropriate range of services for the community and for defining the hospital's mission

- Responsible for the medical ethics practiced within the hospital and the skill level of the medical staff

- Ultimately responsible for the safety of patients

Administration

- Responsible for reducing operating costs to degree possible

- Limits resources without threatening quality of service standards set by physicians and the board

- Responsible for working within regulatory guidelines

- Responsible for meeting payer requirements

- Responsible for developing and implementing efficient and cost effective delivery systems

- Coordinates all hospital services and manages product lines, and personnel

Medical Staff

- Responsible for ordering and providing appropriate medical services

- Encourages additional or changes in resources to meet patient needs in relationship to state of the art medicine

- Responsible for defining quality of services

noted earlier, these are the three principal bodies that drive decisions made and care provided within a hospital. These entities also significantly affect planning for the future. The hospital administration must work with the medical staff to forecast future trends and to recommend and develop short- and long-range strategies concerning how to practice medicine under pending or anticipated government or payer guidelines. As noted earlier, priorities held by the board, the medical staff, and the administration are sometimes very different. As in other highly complex and competitive organizations, solutions to a problem that one group sees as correct may not be seen in the same way by the other groups. Despite this, these groups must function and work together to provide appropriate services for the community at the lowest cost possible.

Decisions regarding strategies and or procedures will often affect these three groups differently, and these differences can generate considerable political activity and tension. But we should appreciate that this tension is in fact necessary for the survival of hospitals: Ideally, it works to force a thorough evaluation of all critical issues, which can lead to the best possible decision for the hospital. However, this is not always the case, which is in part why hospitals are often considered too bureaucratic and slow to make decisions. Still, lack of such ongoing point-counterpoint debates among the members of the triad may lead to the establishment of one-dimensional goals and strategies that will not serve the hospital or the community well. Services that should be provided would not be and vice versa. In most instances, if the members of the triad can identify their common interests, these can serve as a fundamental platform upon which productive debate and discussion can be built and reasonable decisions can be made.

THE EVOLUTION OF ADMINISTRATIVE SKILLS

Hospital administrators, as you will recall, were initially members of the clergy, nurses, and other individuals who had an interest in volunteering their time to help others. Almshouses were the forerunners of today's hospitals and had been managed by people who had no specific training. As time passed, pressures increased to secure more funding to provide more services and to acquire better facilities and equipment; the role of these administrators therefore began to expand to include an additional range of activities that demanded business expertise. Starting in the mid-1800s, government began to take more interest in monitoring these administrators' activities and in making funds available to hospitals, mostly by offering basic health insurance to certain groups. As growing demands for health care services required more predictable sources of revenue, the business aspect of health care began to emerge. As a result, full-time administrators or facility managers were sought to handle operations and the increasing complexity of financing these services.

◄——

▶ **FIGURE 3–5** This illustration provides some insight concerning the balance of political influence that must be maintained in order to initiate and implement programs. Three very different and politically powerful groups must work in concert to provide quality health care at a low cost. These factors, together with the external and internal influences shown earlier, make budgeting and defining strategies for providing health care services to the community a difficult and politically challenging process.

Many religiously affiliated hospitals looked within their organizations for those who had demonstrated leadership and business management qualities. Hospitals without religious affiliations sought individuals who had stronger business backgrounds. Today, hospital administrators are in most cases graduates of business programs. Physicians who are appointed VPs of medical affairs are now selected on the basis not only of their medical knowledge, but also for their management skills and leadership capabilities. Similarly, chairpersons of departments such as medicine, radiology, and pathology are selected with these skills in mind.

THE ADMINISTRATIVE STRUCTURE

Although there is some variation from one hospital to another, most hospitals are organized administratively in fairly similar fashion. Figure 3-6 shows a typical organization chart for a university hospital. Figure 3-7 shows an organization chart of a community hospital.

HOSPITAL EMPLOYEES AND THEIR DEPARTMENTS

A portion of health care industry employment is summarized below:

Health Diagnosing Occupations	Men	Women
Physicians	488	125
Dentists	148	14
Optometrists	18	6
Podiatrists	12	1
	666	146

Health Assessment & Treatment	Men	Women
Registered nurses	103	1703
Pharmacists	123	75
Dieticians	90	9
Therapists	78	303
Respiratory therapists	25	52
Occupational therapists	5	42
Physical therapists	25	80
Speech therapists	6	73
Therapists NEC	10	56
Physician's assistants	20	25
	485	2418

Numbers shown in thousands
Source: U.S. Department of Labor Statistics.

The lion's share of those employed in health care work in hospitals. A unique feature of hospitals is the diversity of training and skills needed to operate these facilities. It has been said of hospitals that they are virtually self-sustaining, needing very few services from the outside. For instance, all hospitals have maintenance departments, which may include architects, project managers, and construction people. These hospital employees could design and construct a new floor for patient care if needed. Also, all hospitals must have efficient and effective hotel management services, needed to change beds and clean patient rooms.

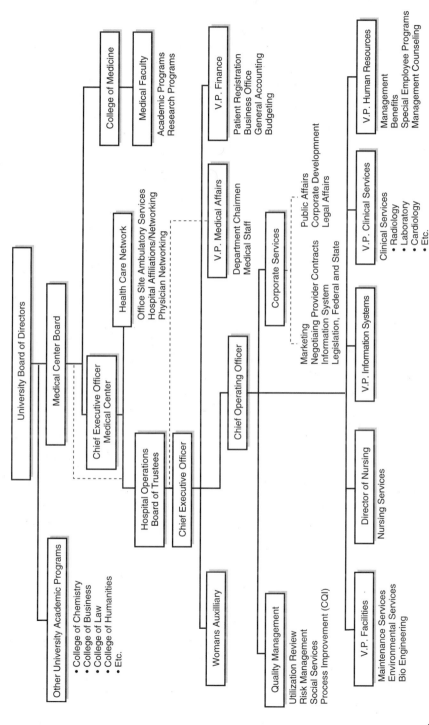

▶ **FIGURE 3–6** A university-based hospital organization structure.

University Board of Directors

Other University Academic Programs
- College of Chemistry
- College of Business
- College of Law
- College of Humanities
- Etc.

Medical Center Board

College of Medicine

Medical Faculty
Academic Programs
Research Programs

Chief Executive Officer
Medical Center

Health Care Network
Office Site Ambulatory Services
Hospital Affiliations/Networking
Physician Networking

V.P. Finance
Patient Registration
Business Office
General Accounting
Budgeting

Hospital Operations
Board of Trustees

Chief Executive Officer

V.P. Medical Affairs
Department Chairmen
Medical Staff

Womans Auxilliary

Chief Operating Officer

Corporate Services
Marketing
Negotiaing Provider Contracts
Information System
Legislation, Federal and State

Public Affairs
Corporate Developmnent
Legal Affairs

Quality Management
Utilization Review
Risk Management
Social Services
Process Improvement (CQI)

V.P. Information Systems

V.P. Clinical Services
Clinical Services
- Radiology
- Laboratory
- Cardiology
- Etc.

V.P. Human Resources
Management
Benefits
Special Employee Programs
Management Counseling

Director of Nursing
Nursing Services

V.P. Facilities
Maintenance Services
Environmental Services
Bio Engineering

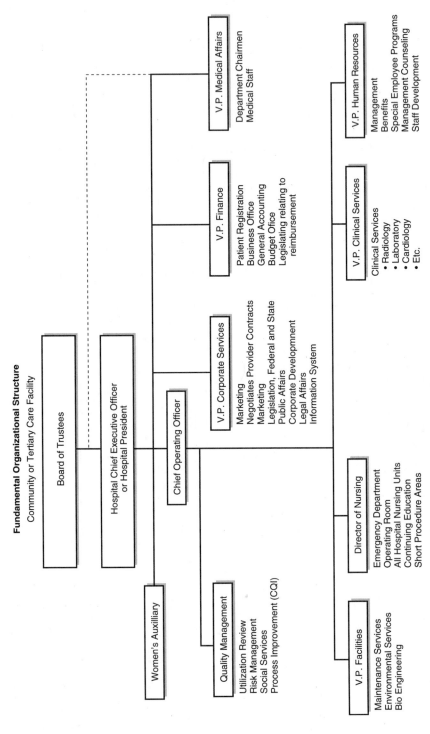

Fundamental Organizational Structure
Community or Tertiary Care Facility

Board of Trustees

Hospital Chief Executive Officer
or Hospital President

Chief Operating Officer

Women's Auxilliary

V.P. Corporate Services
Marketing
Negotiates Provider Contracts
Marketing
Legislation, Federal and State
Public Affairs
Corporate Developmnent
Legal Affairs
Information System

V.P. Finance
Patient Registration
Business Office
General Accounting
Budget Ofice
Legislating relating to
reimbursement

V.P. Medical Affairs
Department Chairmen
Medical Staff

V.P. Human Resources
Management
Benefits
Special Employee Programs
Management Counseling
Staff Development

V.P. Clinical Services
Clinical Services
• Radiology
• Laboratory
• Cardiology
• Etc.

Director of Nursing
Emergency Department
Operating Room
All Hospital Nursing Units
Continuing Education
Short Procedure Areas

Quality Management
Utilization Review
Risk Management
Social Services
Process Improvement (CQI)

V.P. Facilities
Maintenance Services
Environmental Services
Bio Engineering

▶ **FIGURE 3–7** A community or tertiary care hospital organization structure.

Hospitals must also offer a high level of expertise in areas that are often not associated with medical care institutions. For example, hospital dietary services provide a full range of food services and possess specialized knowledge in nutrition. Other capabilities include equipment sterilization and laundry services. Hospital maintenance departments employ skilled service engineers who are responsible for maintaining sophisticated diagnostic and treatment equipment. Other, less well-known departments include internal utilization review and medical records auditing departments. Not only do hospitals need these skills and services, but also they must be immediately available to assure uninterrupted attention to patient care needs. These aspects of hospital operations add to the high cost of running a hospital when compared to other businesses and is one reason why hospitals are so personnel dependent.

No other industry must balance demands from both internal and external elements to the degree that the health care industry must. In addition, the health care industry is unique in that the rapid development of new technologies and procedures leave expensive equipment ineffective before its operational life expectancy is over. Most equipment is likely to become obsolete in five years, which puts tremendous pressures on recapitalization budgets. You will see in Chapter Four how significant this fact is to hospital budgets. It is not uncommon for hospitals to spend 10% of their total budget on equipment-related expenses. Radiology equipment takes up much of this spending.

The effects of current and future legislation add significant uncertainty to capital expenditure decisions. As traditional income streams give way to new and uncertain payment plans, which are being formulated by government and managed care organizations, such decisions are becoming more complex.

A CASE STUDY

Given all these factors, hospital administrations are aggressively looking at how they can begin to position themselves for what the future is most likely to bring. The health care industry is well into its transition from working with fee-for-service agreements based on costs for services provided (retrospective payment) to working with managed care agreements by which full payment is made before the service is provided (prospective payment). The difficulty with many complex transitions is that there is seldom a single point at which all the old elements and influencing factors disappear and the new ones come into full play. Because of this, health care administrators are today trying to function effectively under the requirements of both retrospective and prospective payment agreements, as well as capitation, a difficult balancing act. An example is shown in the following case study.

Because hospitals must become more efficient to operate successfully in the prospective, managed care system of payment, length of stay is being shortened in virtually every hospital in the country. But because many hospitals still receive some fee-for-service payment, adopting an aggressive strategy to reduce length of stay may actually cause a facility to lose money. Attempts to reduce length of stay occur on many fronts. First, physicians must implement patient management plans that can yield shorter stays without reducing quality of care by (1) ordering only those exams that will make a difference, (2) minimizing the number of consulting physicians to the extent possible, and (3) monitoring individual physicians' statistics. Figure 3-8 shows an example of such monitoring. Hospital operations in general must be streamlined to yield as must productivity as possible by (1) ordering exams as soon as possible, (2) performing exams as soon as possible, (3) reducing duplication of services within the facility to the extent possible, and (4) aggressive case management.

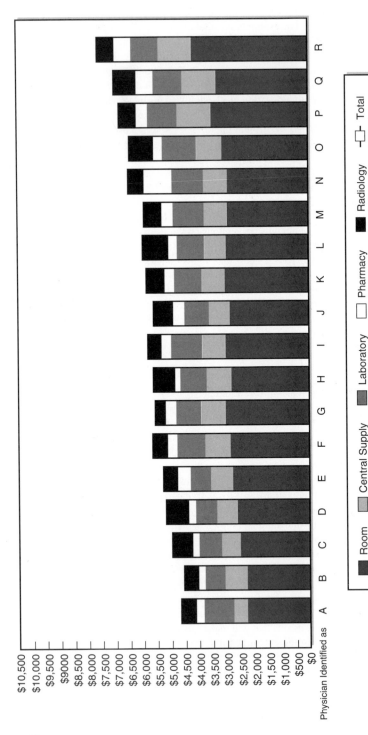

▶ **FIGURE 3–8** As many hospitals are evaluating utilization of resources, how and how often individual physicians order tests is receiving close scrutiny. This chart is a typical summary of the number and type of tests individual physicians have ordered for a large sampling of their patients who have very similar conditions. Each bar represents a physician and shows the tests and relative cost his or her tests generated for the hospital. This "score card" approach provides important information to hospital administrators regarding utilization of the hospital's resources and associated operating costs. It also places significant pressure on physicians to scrutinize every test, procedure, and day of hospital stay they require. This in combination with the risk of malpractice resulting from not ordering appropriate services places the physician in an unenviable position.

DEFINING CRITICAL PATHS

Using critical paths is an operations and patient care strategy that has proven to be very effective for increasing hospital efficiency. Establishing a critical path means that the hospital has evaluated a specific service or treatment and reformulated the manner in which that service will be provided. The goal of a critical path may be to reduce the use of duplicate or unnecessarily expensive medications or to reduce length of stay for patients who are receiving the service. Each facility defines a specific set of goals and benefits for a given critical path. In one example, a case study was conducted to analyze better ways to handle and treat patients who came to the Emergency Department (ED) with pneumonia. The goal was to reduce length of stay by starting the administration of antibiotics as soon as possible. The study found that, on average, antibiotics were not administered until 690 minutes after the patient had been seen by the ED physician. In order to reduce this time, a multidisciplinary group reviewed each step taken prior to the administration of antibiotics.

The group defined a critical path that established an operations plan that involved changing practices by the ED nursing staff, ED physicians, the pharmacy, the radiology department, pathology, and admissions (Figs. 3-9, 3-10, and 3-11). As noted above, the irony is

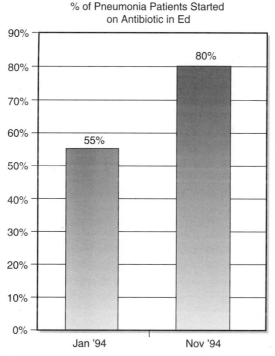

▶ **FIGURE 3-9** Comparison that shows progress made after implementation of a multidisciplinary critical path that involved support from many departments. This graph shows that a much larger percentage of patients received their first dose of antibiotics before they arrived on the nursing floor after implementation. This resulted in more prompt treatment of the patient and less cost to the hospital for the admission because early administration of medications resulted in shorter stays.

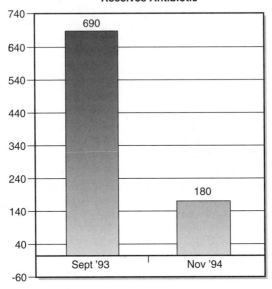

Average Minutes Before Pneumonia Patient Receives Antibiotic

▶ **FIGURE 3–10** Progress of critical path expressed in re-duced-time interval between admission and administration of antibiotics to patients diagnosed with pneumonia.

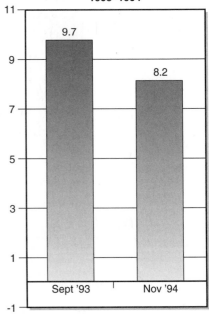

Average LOS for Pneumonia Patients 1993–1994

▶ **FIGURE 3–11** Effect on length of stay of quicker treatment for pneumonia that resulted from developing a critical path team. As a result of this initiative, patients are receiving improved care in the form of quicker treatment, while the hospital gains from a less expensive patient stay.

that some of these patients carry conventional fee-for-service reimbursement coverage, so reducing length of stay for these patients actually reduces the hospital's income. It is impossible ethically and operationally, however, to use two different tracks of care depending on patients' insurance coverage. Clearly, a catch-22 is in place. If operational efficiencies are built into the system too early, revenue is lost. However, it takes time to analyze services and put operational plans in motion. If a facility waits until the balance point between retrospective payment and prospective payment is reached before establishing efficiencies such as critical paths, the institution will lose huge amounts of money because prospective payments will not come close to covering the cost of existing operational inefficiencies. Many hospitals are caught in this dilemma, and the impact to a large part is determined by how fast the market is moving toward capitated contracts. Most hospitals along the East Coast are currently experiencing approximately 12% to 25% capitation.

OPERATIONAL GOALS UNDER FULL CAPITATION

We will see in more detail later that under the old fee-for-service or indemnity payment agreements, such as in the standard Blue Cross plan and commercial payer plans, more activity increased the probability of showing revenue over income. Thus, the more diagnostic tests, treatments, patient days, and occupancy a hospital could shoulder, the better the bottom line was likely to look. This of course varied from hospital to hospital because of payer mix—especially as Blue Cross, commercial, and to some degree Medicare payers represented a greater opportunity for revenue over expenses. However, as the market moves toward capitation, operations at the department and hospital levels are bilaterally affected. Figure 3-12 shows the most fundamental operations elements that may be affected.

A few terms related to capitation need to be clarified initially. *Total lives* defines the number of people who are included in any given contract. It is important for the provider to know what his liability or risk for loss actually is under this contract. Several things affect net risk, but two of the most important are the number and the age of people for whom the provider must provide services under the capitation, or one-time payment, system. *Payment/revenue per month* is the amount of money the provider actually receives for each person who is included in the contract. *Member month* refers to the number of patients for whom the provider is at risk (must provide services to) per month. *Exclusions* are services that the provider is not obligated to provide under the contract. For example, an HMO may contract with a hospital to provide all radiology services except ultrasound and MRI. Or the contract may include *only* MRI or CT; other outpatient imaging will be provided at another facility. Table 3-1 shows one year of activity with a capitated contract for radiology services. Note that the total number of members (people covered by this contract) is 72,000. This represents the *risk,* the number of patients who could receive diagnostic tests per month annualized (number per month × 12). We also see that the revenue this contract will generate is $2.35 per member month (member month × $2.35) Keep in mind that this figure is negotiated between the health care provider and payer. Also keep in mind that the number of visits is irrelevant to revenue. The provider is at risk to provide tests for all patients who come for service and who are covered under this contract based on this revenue formula. The provider will receive no additional funds, even if the number of visits increases. Therefore, increased number of visits is not what the provider wants to see under a capitated contract because as the number of visits increases, the provider's operating costs increase but no additional revenue is received.

Another critical number here is the estimate of *cost per test,* which results from a process referred to as *microcosting.* The provider must know or have a good idea of what its costs

Elements for Consideration	Contract Content, Conditions and Performance Criteria

Impact on Volume and Timeliness of Service	• How many lives are involved
	• What is the range and nature of tests/services covered by contract
	  • Equipment/staff capabilities
	• Requirements for pt wait times for scheduling service
	  • Do services have to be scheduled & performed within a certain period of time?
	• Implications regarding off-hour services
	  • Expectations for weekends & evening hours
	• Exclusions of service
	  • Will volume decrease because of losing a contract?
	  • Which services?
	  • Why?
	• Effect on daily volume
	  • Capacity/capability of equipment, facility, staff

Physician Involvement/ Commitment	• Physician certification issues
	  • For specific procedures
	• Availability of physicians for certain services
	  • Can the physicians' schedule allow us to meet expectations of delay/timeliness criteria?
	• Independent physician contracts
	  • Separate provider contracts that impact "hospital" services
	  • Special billing procedures to CCH from physician provider contracts directly with payer
	• Validating physician eligibility under contract
	  • Will payer recognize ordering physician as being appropriate for the service requested?
	• Will contract exclude participation of certain physicians?
	  • Will this affect physician availability?
	  • Will only certain physicians be able to participate?

Reporting Requirements	• Expectation for turnaround time • Does the report/service have to be available within a certain time frame? • Expectations for providing payer with documentation (i.e., copies of reports)

▶ **FIGURE 3–12** Indicates the various operations that are affected as hospitals enter into contracts with managed care organizations. Immediate implications involve a more complex screen of information during scheduling, patient registration, and physician certification.

Preregistration and Scheduling Criteria	• Linking study ordered with charge master
	    • Compatibility of language/terms used for the service
	• Defining pt. eligibility for service under the contract
	• Verifying procedures entered into system are compatible with patient's contract
	    • We must avoid doing cases outside payer contracts
	• Expectations about the type of precertification documentation CCH must forward to payer
	    • Which physician may order the study/service under the contract?
	    • Verify the service ordered is within CCH's contract
	• Impact on flexibility of scheduling other "noncontract" services

▶ **FIGURE 3–12** *Continued*

are for each service it is under contract to provide. In this example, the average cost of all exams provided under this contract in aggregate is estimated to be $126,000, plus radiologists' charges to interpret studies. (Under such an agreement, the radiologists will not bill separately for their interpretation, but will be paid by the hospital from the revenue the hospital gets from the per member month formula.) In this example, the radiology income from this contract is $15,000. The remainder is revenue over expenses, or *profit*. As you will see later, there are many indirect expenses that must be accounted for in this contract as well. Examples are heat, electricity, and insurance. Table 3-2 shows an example of microcosting a particular study. This per exam cost must be added to the hospital's indirect expenses to get an average per exam cost. The accuracy of these cost accounting calculations obviously determines the accuracy of the net income figure that appears in Table 3-1. Many hospitals and departments do not understand their actual per exam costs. Clearly, such an understanding will have to be improved substantially as capitation becomes a bigger part of a hospital's revenue stream. It is interesting to note that if a provider has a group of patients of 20,000 in a capitated contract, the provider realizes financial gains if no patients come for services. The reason is that as services are rendered operating costs increase. The income remains constant from the HMO regardless of the number of patients who are served.

From this example, one can also see why administrators are anxious to reduce operating costs associated with inpatient activity, for example, average length of stay, total patient days, and average cost per admission (DRG specific). Other potential operational efficiencies involve staffing levels, and administrators are wrestling with ways to keep staffing as flexible as possible as they monitor the number of FTEs (Full-Time Equivalent) employee per occupied bed. In fact, as you will see later in the text, as a result of establishing a critical path for DRG 209 (hip surgery), the average length of stay was reduced from 8.74 days in 1993 to 6.63 days in 1994. General opinion that quality of care remained constant or may actually have improved slightly (Figs. 3-13 and 3-14). A single critical path effort can have

▶ TABLE 3–1
CALCULATING NET MONTHLY INCOME BASED ON MANAGED CARE CONTRACT (Hypothetical)

NUMBER OF MEMBERS COVERED PER MONTH	ANNUAL REVENUE	REVENUE/MONTH	PATIENT VISITS	ESTIMATED (OPERATING) COST	M.D. FEES	TOTAL COST	HOSPITAL'S PROFIT/LOSS
72,000	$1,680,000	$140,000	1440	$126,000	$15,000	$135,000	$5,000

One can see from this simplified illustration how net revenue managed care contracts are tracked by hospital administrators Clearly, there is no longer a relationship between traditional charges and what is actually collected.

▶ TABLE 3−2
EXAMINATION COST ANALYSIS FOR ULTRASOUND PROCEDURE

Direct Costs		
Supplies		
Film 4 8×10	$8.00	
Processing chem (4 sheets of film)	$0.25	
Electricity film processor	$0.25	
Gel/lubricant	$0.35	
4×4 gauze pads	$0.15	
Film jacket (new patients)	$3.00	
Request form and miscellaneous paper supplies	$4.00	
Miscellaneous forms/sub folders	$2.00	
		$18.00
Salaries		
Technologist (30 min)	$8.50	
Escort (in pts) 25 min. Transportation	$4.25	
Receptionist & Scheduling (20 min.)	$6.20	
File Clerk (20 min.)	$6.20	
Transcript (10 min. typing & miscellaneous handling	$2.00	
	$27.15	
Cost of benefits (Cal. @ 30%)	$8.15	$35.30
Indirect Costs		
Utilities Building, Heating, Water, Electricity		
Insurance, maintenance, etc.		
Building Depreciation (over 20 yrs)		
Annual average cost sq/ft	$150.00	
Size of associated space (sq. ft)	×300	
Total Cost/year	$2,250.00	
Number of exams performed/year	3500	
Indirect cost per/exam		$0.64
Cost of Equipment per Exam		
Number of exams performed per year	3500	
Equipment Life 6 Years	×6	
Total Exams Performed	21,000	
Estimated Purchase Price	$450,000	$21.43
Other Minor Equipment Costs per Exam		
Estimated accumulated purchase price	$5,000	$0.24
		$75.60

An example of how cost per exam can be defined. A defined example of cost exam analysis is commonly referred to as microcosting. The finance department can provide figures to be used for overhead (indirect costs).

a positive affect in other ways. Figure 3-1 shows the improved patient management procedures implemented for DRG is 209 carried over in other DRGs to yield positive changes there as well.

Besides the financial risks and conditions involved in capitation contracts, operational initiatives need to be addressed strenuously, as shown in Figure 3-12, a summary of contract elements and operational performance criteria that must be in place and compatible with each other.

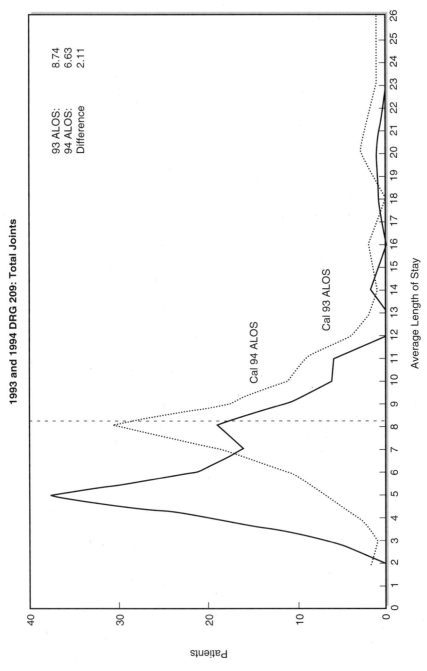

1993 and 1994 DRG 209: Total Joints

93 ALOS: 8.74
94 ALOS: 6.63
Difference   2.11

Cal 94 ALOS

Cal 93 ALOS

Patients

Average Length of Stay

▶ **FIGURE 3–13**   Results of establishing a single critical path.

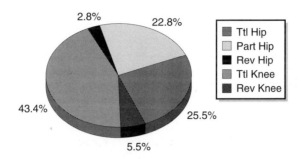

Other Procedures Affected by DRG 209

DRG 209: FY 93 and FY 94 Comparison

	Cal 1993	Cal 1994	
	ALOS	ALOS	ALOS Chg
Ttl Hip	8.92	5.91	-3.01
Part Hip	9.03	8.54	-0.49
Rev Hip	10.00	6.75	-3.25
Ttl Knee	8.37	6.00	-2.37
Rev Knee	7.00	4.75	-2.25
TOTAL	8.74	6.63	-2.11

▶ **FIGURE 3-14** Other benefits can result from implementing a single critical path.

STUDY QUESTIONS

1. Give three examples that indicate the size of the health care industry.
2. List two external influences on each of the activities below that significantly affect decisions made by key hospital administrators.
   a. Making capital budget decisions
   b. Making changes in mission
   c. Developing new services
3. List two internal influences that significantly affect the decisions hospital administrators make regarding policy and budget (capital or operating).
4. Distinguish between these categories of hospital structure: (1) public, (2) private not-for-profit, (2) private for-profit. How should net revenue after expenses be handled by these organizations in order to maintain their current corporate status?
5. Describe the responsibilities of the board of directors, its composition, and its membership selection criteria.
6. What landmark cases helped to define the responsibilities of boards regarding quality of care and safety of patients?

7. What is the relationship between a community and a private not-for-profit community hospital? Address such issues as

   cost of service,
   scope of service provided/needed, and
   assessment of needs for service.

8. Briefly describe the structure of the medical staff in a hospital and who governs its members and how.

9. Explain the political and economic difficulties that exist between the board, the administration, and the medical staff. In what ways do you think the missions and objectives of these groups differ?

10. In what ways is the medical staff and the hospital administration dependent on each other? If you were a hospital administrator, what would you do to make this relationship positive? In turn, what would you expect the medical staff to do?

FOUR

Financial Aspects of Hospital Management

OBJECTIVES FOR STUDY

After reading this chapter, the student will

- ▶ Understand the role of the chief financial officer.

- ▶ Appreciate the need for various budgets and the need to monitor variances from the budget.

- ▶ Understand the basic steps that must be taken to develop the operating and capital budgets.

- ▶ Appreciate the need for a mission statement, how this document affects the setting of budget goals, and how projects for new or expanded services are evaluated.

- ▶ Understand the nature of the various types of budgets.

- ▶ Understand the concept of capital depreciation.

- ▶ Understand how and why outside influences affect a hospital's mission statement and eventually affect how capital funds will be distributed within the hospital.

- ▶ Appreciate the various tools used by hospital financial managers to monitor the financial status of the hospital.

- ▶ Appreciate the appropriateness of defining specific product lines that hospitals offer patients to improve future revenue.

- ▶ Understand the basic factors involved in hospital affiliations and buyouts and how these can affect a hospital's financial picture.

- ▶ Appreciate how a hospital's mission statement can be influenced by legislation.

▶ Understand why the application of strong business policies and philosophies is necessary in order for hospitals to stay solvent in today's health care environment.

INTRODUCTION

In the past, the delivery of health care was often accomplished primarily as charity. The major emphasis was on providing services, and the managers of early health care facilities hoped that some payment would be given in return. Health care delivery systems developed slowly through the early 1800s, but accelerated quickly throughout the rest of the century and into the 1900s. As we noted in the previous chapters, this growth eventually required more sophisticated financial and accounting methods in order to monitor income, manage present funds, and search for new funds so future demands for health care services could be met. Fledgling institutions continued to grow and attract new patients as insurance programs provided more based their reimbursements. To help drive this growth, growing practices hired more and more highly skilled physicians. Well-known and energetic physicians who could provide advanced services were aggressively recruited by those facilities whose missions placed them in leadership positions for meeting future health care needs.

HOSPITAL-BASED HEALTH CARE SERVICES IS BIG BUSINESS

Government regulation of health care is directly connected to hospitals' acceptance of government funding. As the amount of health care-related legislation continued to increase, increasing funds made available through grants and low interest loans encouraged hospitals to adopt new and more effective accounting and financial systems.

The evolution of the application of strong and sophisticated accounting and financial systems to hospital management decisions came slowly, however. In fact, it is the view of many that the development of such financial expertise has lagged many years behind the accelerated pace of overall patient activity and demand for services. Probably, there were two major reasons for this. The first was that health care was not viewed as principally a business. There was, and in many cases still is, resistance to moving away from the industry's strong roots as a provider of vital life and health services to the community and toward a strong business posture. The roots of hospital services go back through a long lineage of almshouses and charitable facilities managed mostly by volunteers whose mission was to provide service first and then to look for funding. Later, the federal government implemented plans that encouraged treatment of the poor by making special provisions to reimburse expenses for such medical services. This heritage meant that most hospitals felt obligated to provide services when payment was due but not forthcoming. All these elements contributed to the practice of *cost accounting* procedures to measure the current position of a hospital. Using proactive business approaches that encouraged bottom-line oriented decisions was often considered inappropriate. In fact, many community hospitals until perhaps the 1940s or 1950s defined their financial goal as *not* generating excess revenue over expenses, but rather as maintaining just enough income over expenses to cover emergencies. Money needed for future building or program needs was to come from fund drives, the community, and philanthropists.

THE BUDGET: WHY?

If there is enough money coming into the hospital to cover expenses, why not simply earmark a certain amount for future growth each year and ask your managers, directors, and administrators to use their creative energies and skills to cut costs wherever possible? In addition, why not rely on their good judgment leading them to buy only the equipment and supplies that are actually needed? If there are funds left over at the end of the year after these operations expenditures, they can be added to the money that has already been earmarked for future program needs. It sounds like a plan to me! This plan, however, has one or two fundamental flaws. Not everybody views "cut costs where possible" in the same way, and relying on "creative energy and skill" to cut costs can easily translate into generating new and even greater expenses for the institution. There are surely more than two fundamental flaws in our plan, but the two noted above demonstrate that financial management based primarily on good intent and human self-discipline can lead to trouble, if not to financial ruin. This is particularly true in the highly political environment in which hospitals must function. In addition, history shows that humans are generally not very good at self-denial. Therefore, the only way to insure financial success is to develop a firm but realistic budget—in effect a blueprint for spending and saving and give all managers accountability for following the blueprint.

THE FUNCTION OF A BUDGET

There are several basic functions that the budget process serves:

1. Channels funds for specific use within the facility
2. Helps prevent unnecessary spending
3. Provides a measure of effectiveness of services
4. Helps set management and operational goals
5. Helps assure adherence to the facility's mission
6. Helps evaluate management performance
7. Helps force development of alternative operating plans
8. Helps management analyze percentage of effort and return
9. Provides a blueprint to help assess day to day operations
10. Forces an analysis of fund allocation for services
11. Helps evaluate effective services on a per cost basis
12. Provides an opportunity to evaluate organizational goals and to define strategies
13. Provides an opportunity to answer the question, What changes in operations do we plan to make to correct identified operational and fiscal problems?

Budgets provide a structure or plan for spending. Also, budgets are approved by someone or by a group of individuals who function at a distance from everyday activities, which is vital to the setting of goals and objectives. In a hospital setting, those who create the fundamental rules for allocating money and provide parameters to department directors are the board of directors, the chief financial officer, and senior administrators. These people essentially operate as a unit to construct the budgeting process and to define strategies. They establish requirements that will govern how funds are distributed throughout the institution. They also determine such things as which clinical programs will be considered for new funding; the rate of across-the-board salary adjustments for employees; and which major building, renovation, or service programs will be funded.

Once a budget is in place, it is very important for a hospital to establish standards for performance against which patient activity, cost, and the budget can be evaluated. Such standards can be seen as the hospital's vital signs. A sample of one hospital's vital signs are listed below. These vital signs relate to standards for institutional performance, which can be viewed as operational imperatives. These operational imperatives form a blueprint for daily operations and decision making in concert with the institution's overall strategy.

Operational Vital Signs
Admissions
Average length of stay
Patient days
Average daily census
Overall activity of outpatient services
Overall staffing based on defined inpatient and outpatient activity

THE MISSION AND VISION STATEMENT

There is an element that is absolutely essential to the budgeting process and that is the mission or vision statement of the hospital. In some respects, the institution's mission statement is a miniconstitution rolled into one paragraph; it is sometimes elaborated in a more expansive document of two or three pages. The mission statement is approved by the board of directors and becomes the beacon that guides all strategic planning. It provides direction to the institution's medical staff because it controls the level of technology that will be available and the type and scope of clinical programs that will be supported. The mission statement is developed by the senior administration, but it must be approved by the board.

The content of mission statements can vary considerably from hospital to hospital. Their mission statements may set one hospital on a campaign to develop a high-tech, high-expense trauma service and lead another facility *not* to proceed in that direction. Figures 4-1 and 4-2 show two mission statements and a summary of guiding principles that will support a hospitals mission statement. The difference in the nature and scope of medical care provided by these two institutions is very evident.

The scope of service described in a mission statement is not an indication of the quality of services that are provided. In fact, patients can often point to institutions that have less grandiose mission statements but are held in higher regard for the quality of service they

---

VISION STATEMENT

Hospital will be recognized as a dedicated, community-based health care organization which enjoys integrated provider relationships that foster excellence in clinical care and personal service. It will seek to develop and implement programs and services which will enhance the health status of the community. The Hospital will strive to exceed the expectations of those it serves, maintain standards of the highest quality, and promote a rewarding work environment.

▶ **FIGURE 4-1** A vision statement that helps set strategies and service initiatives for an organization.

GUIDING PRINCIPLES

Mission – To preserve the charitable, community-based mission of The Hospital.

Governance – To maintain a local, voluntary, committed and innovative governing body which reflects the community's commitment to supporting high quality, fiscally responsible medical services.

Quality of Care – To ensure a standard of care and personal attention which meets the needs of our patients, community, employees, and physicians.

Community Relationship – To preserve a strong commitment to and relationship with the community.

Employees – To provide a challenging and rewarding environment where employees are encouraged to grow personally and professionally, thereby adding to the overall benefit and adaptability of the organization as it seeks to meet the needs of the community.

Physical plant – To maintain a modern facility which preserves the charm, historical significance and heritage of citizens.

Relationships with Other Providers – To seek alliances with other health care providers and community resources which have a common set of values and which would enhance and ensure The Hospital's present and future commitment to the individuals it serves. These relationships should assist and encourage us to maintain the unique character of our vision while enabling us to meet the challenges of the future.

Organizational Culture – To foster relationships of trust throughout the organization which are based on open communication and a spirit of collaboration, cooperation and respect.

▶ **FIGURE 4-2** Important concepts that are identified in order to support an institution's defined mission.

provide than facilities whose mission is to be at the leading edge of technology. Once a mission statement is written, it generally remains unchanged for several years. This provides the administration with stability so that midrange strategies can be evaluated and developed. In this fashion, mission statements are translated into specific programs and quantified into annual budgets. Using the mission statement as a guide, hospital financial officers and administrators budget funds through two main channels, the operating budget and the capital budget.

THE OPERATING BUDGET

Basic elements of a hospital's operating budget are shown in Figure 4-3. This management tool focuses on the amount and distribution of funds needed to support everyday operational expenses. Each item identified in the budget is referred to as a line item. You will note from looking at Figure 4-3(B) that the personnel budget is a major part of the operating budget. Because of its complexity and because personnel expenses are calculated differently from commodities expenses, the personnel budget is developed separately and lat-

BASIC ELEMENTS OF A HOSPITAL BUDGET

Direct Expenses
Operating budget
  Salaries
  Benefits
  Drugs, other pharmaceutical
    needs
  Supplies
  Minor equipment
  Miscellaneous minor
    expenses
Advertising/marketing
Leases/rentals
Discretionary expenses
Other direct expenses
Bad debt/discounts

Indirect Expenses
Building depreciation
Equiment depreciation
Heat/light/telephone, etc.
  (utilities)
Building Maintenance
Service contracts
Purchased services/consultants

Revenue
Operating income from principal services
Other operating income
Nonoperating income/investments

Funds
Various fund balances from such
  accounts as:
  Grants/gifts from donors and
    philanthropy
  Building funds
  Dedicated funds defined by donor

A

Community Hospital Expenditures, 1992

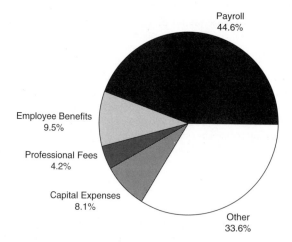

Payroll 44.6%

Employee Benefits 9.5%

Professional Fees 4.2%

Capital Expenses 8.1%

Other 33.6%

B

▶ **FIGURE 4–3** (A) Basic elements of a hospital's operating budget. (B) Overall distribution of expenses. Note the portion of overall expenses that are consumed by personnel and benefit expenses. In most hospitals, employee benefits add 25% to 30% to basic salary. An employee may estimate the total compensation by adding benefit costs to the basic hourly rate.

er combined with the overall operating budget. The personnel expense component of the operating budget includes such line items as benefits, Social Security contributions, overtime, and health insurance.

In addition to personnel expenses, the operating budget has other major components which are sometimes referred to as commodities expenses. Also, service expenses of several types appear in the hospital's operating budget. Utility costs for heating, water, and electricity are significant. Electricity, for example, for a 250-bed facility will approach $1 million annually. Another group of line items is known as discretionary expenses, expenses which are generally considered to be nonessential in the sense that they can be frozen or dissolved without having an immediate impact on quality or efficiency of operations. Examples of discretionary expenses are travel expenses, library expenses, tuition reimbursements, and other educational/inservice expenses. When budget cuts begin, discretionary expenses are often the first line items to be reduced or cut altogether. Line items in the operating budget can also be broken into expenses fixed and variable expenses. The concepts of fixed and variable expenses will be discussed in detail later.

THE CAPITAL BUDGET AND DEPRECIATION EXPENSES

The capital budget is very different from the operating budget, but as we will see later, they are linked to one another. The typical criteria for identifying a purchase as a capital item, as opposed to an operating expense, is that it must have a cost of $2000 or more and must have a life expectancy of at least three years. Although this seems fairly straightforward, institutions differ as to how they define certain capital budget items. In general, though, the capital budget focuses on expenditures made to support items that have a relatively long life and are relatively expensive. Examples are X-ray equipment and building renovations.

As equipment depreciates in value, this declining value is viewed by accountants as an expense. In for-profit industries, part of this expense is returned to the business through tax deductions.

Equipment Depreciation Calculations

R/F X-ray machine

Year purchased	Cost	Estimated life	Annual depreciation	Year fully depreciated
1993	$435,000	8 yrs	$54,475	2001

CAPITAL EROSION

Capital erosion is an important concept to understand because it affects planning for acquisition of new equipment. It refers to the combined effect of inflation of prices for future equipment and the continually depreciating value of existing equipment (Table 4-1). Thus, each piece of equipment purchased carries not only the immediate acquisition cost, but also future costs associated with its replacement.

As noted above, the capital and operating budgets are very dependent on each other despite the fact that they represent very different items and are developed in very different manners. For example, one should not consider budgeting for an additional piece of capital equipment unless consideration is given to associated expenses, such as depreciation, supplies, and personnel expenses, that will fall into the operating budget.

▶ TABLE 4−1
ESTIMATED USEFUL LIFE OF IMAGING EQUIPMENT

DESCRIPTION	YEARS
Radiographic/fluoroscopic machine	8
Ultrasound scanner	5
Radiographic machine	8
Therapy accelerator	7
CT scanner	5
MRI scanner	5

Purchase price, 1990 R/F machine	EXAMPLE OF CAPITAL EROSION 1998 Replacement cost	1998 Trade-in value	Net increase in cost
$375,000	$450,372	$10,000	$65,372

Illustrates the concept of capital erosion. Keeping a healthy capital fund is vital to a hospital's well-being. This is particularly true today, as many hospitals are not generating enough funds from regular operations to support expensive equipment purchases and renovation projects.

WHICH COMES FIRST, THE CHICKEN OR THE EGG? (CAPITAL OR OPERATING EXPENSES)

The capital budget actually drives the operating budget to a large degree. Capital expenditures are an important part of any institution's overall financial program because they not only create significant debt (mortgages), but also generate secondary costs in the form of interest payments to lending institutions or bond holders, which are operating budget items. However, without capital expenses, no, or very few, services could be provided. Therefore, to some degree, one can gauge the mission of a hospital by the size and composition of its capital assets. The capital budget will contain funds for renovations and upgrades to the existing plant or for the building of a proposed new facility. Other items in the capital budget include emergency generators, electrical switch gear for the hospital's electric and telephone systems, and the heating and air conditioning (HVAC) systems. One of the most important capital budget decisions an administrator can make is to determine whether it is more prudent to build a new facility or to renovate an existing one.

Hospitals have recouped depreciation losses from Medicare and other payer reimbursements. However, these reimbursements are one of the casualties of health care reform. In the past, up to 80% of depreciation expenses were reimbursed. Today, the amount of reimbursement is almost zero. Calculating depreciation is still important for an institution's own business plan. In theory, money that relates to depreciated expenses should be kept in a designated fund and reinvested so that it will grow and can be used to pay for replacement equipment or buildings in the future.

CALCULATING DEPRECIATION OF ASSETS

Depreciation is calculated on the basis of equipment life spans, which are listed in various tables. *Depreciated life* refers to the estimated time a piece of equipment will be reasonably current and to its mechanical life or durability. Buildings are considered to be fully depreciated after 25 or 30 years. However, pieces of equipment within that building have different depreciation values. A routine diagnostic X-ray machine may have a depreciation life of 12 years, while an ultrasound scanner's life expectancy is only 6 years. In theory, this means that after 12 years the X-ray machine is significantly less useful in providing current services and should be replaced. Table 4-1 shows the depreciation lives for different capital items. We will see when we discuss radiology administration how depreciation and other financial considerations are used when estimating the efficacy of a new clinical program.

BUDGETING VARIOUS ACCOUNTS

Budgets are defined and used to monitor many different accounts. A budget is a managing tool that tracks funds that have been allocated for a specific type or group of expenses. Hospitals develop and manage many different accounts, which have their own budgets. Some of these accounts are:

- Revenue
- Allowances
- Cash
- Depreciation

THE BUDGET CYCLE

All facilities have a budget management period, which is often referred to as a budget cycle or fiscal year. The fiscal year for the federal government, for example, begins each October 1 and ends September 30. Some businesses use the calendar year, January 1 through December 31, but many use July 1 through June 30.

In many hospitals, the budget process generally requires approximately four months to complete, with the clock starting when the board of directors approves the final financial goals and strategies for the hospital for the coming year. Worksheets are prepared and sent to department directors with instructions. The basic steps are described schematically in Figure 4-4. Some facilities have adopted very cumbersome regimens, while others have used rather streamlined procedures. If a facility operates on July 1 fiscal cycle, department directors will usually receive their budget packets in February or March. Final board approval should occur in May or early June and implementation begin July 1.

WHO IS INVOLVED IN THE BUDGET PROCESS?

As noted above, several different groups and management levels within an organization participate is completing budgets after the board of directors approves the financial criteria and goals for the coming year. The board dictates through its interpretation of the hospital's mission how much total revenue can be expected and what the overall allocation of those funds will be for the coming year. More specifically, it will determine how much will go to capital expenditures, savings, contingency expenses, and new programs and services. This includes approving plans for building new services, such as a trauma or neonatal service. Funds requested by department directors to expand existing services are also evaluated against the hospital's fiscal goals.

FORMULATING EXPENSES

As the budget is being developed, several sources offer ideas for new hospital programs, services, buildings, and research endeavors which are considered for approval through the

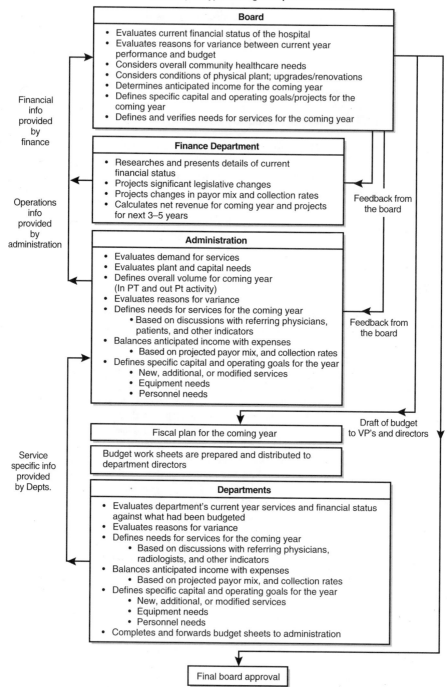

Summary of Typical Budget Preparation Process

Board
- Evaluates current financial status of the hospital
- Evaluates reasons for variance between current year performance and budget
- Considers overall community healthcare needs
- Considers conditions of physical plant; upgrades/renovations
- Determines anticipated income for the coming year
- Defines specific capital and operating goals/projects for the coming year
- Defines and verifies needs for services for the coming year

Financial info provided by finance

Finance Department
- Researches and presents details of current financial status
- Projects significant legislative changes
- Projects changes in payor mix and collection rates
- Calculates net revenue for coming year and projects for next 3–5 years

Feedback from the board

Operations info provided by administration

Administration
- Evaluates demand for services
- Evaluates plant and capital needs
- Defines overall volume for coming year (In PT and out Pt activity)
- Evaluates reasons for variance
- Defines needs for services for the coming year
  - Based on discussions with referring physicians, patients, and other indicators
- Balances anticipated income with expenses
  - Based on projected payor mix, and collection rates
- Defines specific capital and operating goals for the year
  - New, additional, or modified services
  - Equipment needs
  - Personnel needs

Feedback from the board

Fiscal plan for the coming year

Budget work sheets are prepared and distributed to department directors

Draft of budget to VP's and directors

Service specific info provided by Depts.

Departments
- Evaluates department's current year services and financial status against what had been budgeted
- Evaluates reasons for variance
- Defines needs for services for the coming year
  - Based on discussions with referring physicians, radiologists, and other indicators
- Balances anticipated income with expenses
  - Based on projected payor mix, and collection rates
- Defines specific capital and operating goals for the year
  - New, additional, or modified services
  - Equipment needs
  - Personnel needs
- Completes and forwards budget sheets to administration

Final board approval

▶ **FIGURE 4–4** The complexity of the budget process varies considerably among hospitals. This illustration, however, traces a process that is common to many institutions.

budget process. Requests may come from the community. Business leaders may join together either as concerned individual citizens or in formal organizations to generate political clout to promote specific community health care needs. They will suggest to hospital administrators or to board members that a new service needs to be added or an existing service must be improved, expanded, or perhaps deleted. They may also work to discourage a hospital from moving ahead with plans that they think might be too expensive for the community.

Another source of input is the medical staff, which may make suggestions for new or expanded programs. These suggestions can carry considerable weight. Certainly, hospital administrators provide very significant input and counsel. The chief financial officer has a substantial role in defining the upcoming year's budget. His or her job is not only to keep an eye on the hospital's current financial conditions, but also to watch upcoming legislation and payer trends. This information is vital because any new program being considered by the hospital administration must be appropriate and offer payment under future regulations.

Below are some fundamental planning questions that need to be considered before developing budget goals and criteria for the coming year.

1. How much capital funding do we need to support programs next year and over the next five years?
2. What will the source of funding be for these investments?
3. Over what time period do we spend what percentage of these allocated funds?
4. What plans do we have in place to generate more income?
5. Are we setting aside enough money to replace existing capital assets (i.e., equipment and buildings)?
6. How much revenue can we anticipate over the coming year?
7. What return do we expect on our capital investments?
8. When will we begin to see some of this return?
9. What role will our medical staff play in generating new income from new or expanded services made possible by the hospital's purchase of equipment, new buildings, and services?

PUTTING IT TOGETHER

The board compiles such information in the initial stages of the budget process and sometimes assigns research duties to various subcommittees. You may recall our earlier discussion about the makeup and function of the board of directors and about the importance of having people with various expertise on the subcommittees working on different aspects of budget development. Remember also the discussion in Chapter Three regarding internal and external influencing factors.

Once general decisions regarding the major programs the board will support in the coming year are complete, detailed guidelines and worksheets are prepared and forwarded to department heads throughout the hospital. The department directors must complete the worksheets and return them to the hospital's accounting department, or in some cases to the administration, for initial review. As we will see later, it is each department's responsibility to follow much the same process the hospital uses to help identify operating and capital expenditures for the department. Department equipment needs are formalized by requests for new or expanded programs which are defined, developed, and proposed by department directors and their chairpersons. These are rolled into the various worksheets with appropriate support information and handed back to the hospital administration for consideration and approval.

COMMUNITY ASSESSMENT OF AND INPUT TO MAJOR PROGRAMS

There is always the question of how the community may view a hospital's proposed plans for expansion or the development of major new services. This question looms larger in community hospitals than in large facilities that are located in urban areas or than in university-based facilities. It is therefore extremely important that board members, administrators, and physicians keep in close touch with community leaders who can in turn keep the community informed as the hospital proposed new programs. Failing to do so can be disastrous. In some instances, hospitals have promoted worthwhile and cost-effective programs only to have them receive strong negative community reaction because of a lack of understanding on the part of the business community or the general population.

We must keep in mind that a good portion of a hospital's expenses are paid by businesses that pay health insurance premiums for their employees. Thus, community sentiment among business leaders can run very high for or against a proposed hospital building program. The business community may believe that a program proposed by a hospital will unnecessarily increase use of health care services. As we have seen previously, availability of services does indeed encourage demand for them and increase health costs. The hospital must therefore get direction from its mission statement to help assure that its proposal is appropriate for the community.

In summary, a hospital budget cannot be developed in a vacuum. Both internal and external influences must be considered. What services a hospital provides and how it provides them is of high interest to the community. The trend today is to flatten or decrease hospital spending. However, not delivering worthwhile new services to a community can seriously impede a facility's ability to meet future health care needs and to fulfill its obligation to the community. A balance must be struck between developing new and improved services and holding costs to a minimum. A balance that worried health care managers from the very beginning, demand for services and limited reimbursement.

THE MONTHLY BUDGET VARIANCE REPORT

Although it is very important for an organization to develop a budget, it is equally important to follow expenses during the year and to measure them against what had been budgeted. This process is perhaps one of the most disliked and cumbersome aspects of management. There are several reasons for this, not the least of which is the feeling of continuous pressure and anxiety it evokes among department directors and their supervisors. Also, surprisingly poor and inefficient financial monitoring systems are often used to match actual expenses against the budget. This certainly makes the job of comparing actual expenses with the budget even more difficult.

Tracking expenses is very cumbersome. Each department must work in close coordination to assure that all the necessary elements of information needed for budget tracking are in place and available when needed. This is not always an easy task. For example, suppose that a case of needles was ordered on the 15th of the month. Depending on when and how accurately the request was transcribed into a purchase order (PO) by the purchasing department and how quickly the PO was forwarded to the supplier, the expense may or may not be logged as an expense that the department anticipated and budgeted for. If the supplier does not have the item in stock, it will be delivered later than anticipated and also expensed in the wrong time period; significant budget variances are therefore likely to result. If the order is cancelled, proper credit may not be given back to the department and this will influence how budget variances are recorded.

These and many other possibilities can cause considerable accounting and budget tracking problems. Suppose that the accounting department made an error and logged the item to the wrong department. As a result, a department's expenses can show a month's expenses to be either too high or under budget, and this results in unnecessary heartburn for all involved. If we consider the number of items, that are ordered in any given month by a department, we can see why the effort needed to reconcile the department's monthly budget variance report can be hair-raising (Table 4-2).

After department directors complete their monthly variance reports and explanations of variances, they send them to hospital administrators for review and then on to the accounting department so that corrections and adjustments can be entered into the final monthly or quarterly variance report. The variance report is reviewed by the chief financial officer and the board of directors.

ACCRUED EXPENSES

Another complication involved in tracking budget variances comes in the form of accrued expenses. Accruing expenses is a common practice and occurs when the accounting department prelogs an expense in anticipation that charges will occur in the future. This is a banking procedure on the expense side of the budget that is practiced by almost every organization to some degree. Accrued expenses are sometimes used for items, such as service contracts, that have a single annual charge. This charge is sometimes broken into monthly expenses.

Accrued expenses can indeed complicate budget variance reporting. For example, the annual fee for a service contract can change dramatically in the middle of the year. In other instances, accrued expenses if not monitored carefully can give a falsely favorable monthly bottom line to a department's budget: If overspending on a certain line occurs, accrued expenses could help the department's budget look fine for that month. The opposite is also true: If money that has been designated for an accrued item is spent sooner than initially expected, the bottom line will likely look unfavorable.

In summary, accurately monitoring actual expenses against the budget is very dependent on accurate hospital accounting, well-developed and timely supply ordering procedures, and finely tuned hospital expense tracking systems. Some recommended practices are outlined below:

1. Purchasing supplies at the lowest price possible
2. Linking the timeliness of placing orders with delivery and billing
3. Placing reasonable controls on purchase requisitions
4. Possessing a thorough understanding of hospital accrual systems
5. Keeping inventory as low as possible
6. Reviewing carefully monthly charges entered against departments

114

▶ TABLE 4–2
MONTHLY VARIANCE REPORT

CURRENT MONTH				Expense Line Items	YEAR TO DATE			
Actual	Budget	Variance	% Var		Actual	Budget	Variance	% Var
$194,140	$182,759	$11,381	6.23%	100 Salaries	$1,620,430	$1,523,370	$107,477	7.06%
$68,653	$48,350	$20,303	41.99%	390 Medical Supplies	$515,342	$435,151	$90,608	20.82%
($118,450)	$39,375	($157,826)	−400.82%	395 Film & Processing	$239,414	$354,374	($104,542)	−29.50%
$6,174	$4,911	$1,262	25.70%	460 Office Supplies	$41,450	$44,202	$7,666	17.34%
$3,200	$957	$2,242	234.27%	490 Minor Equip	$15,655	$8,604	$17,468	203.03%
$0	$0	$0	ERR	500 Uniforms & Scrubs	$0	$0	$10,417	0.00%
$17,280	$26,409	($9,129)	−34.57%	560 Service Contracts	$201,531	$237,678	($25,731)	−10.83%
$79,535	$10,125	$69,410	685.53%	570 Repairs & Maintenance	$308,250	$91,125	$227,542	249.70%
$16,920	$7,020	$9,900	141.02%	600 Purchased Services	$538,542	$406,620	$142,339	35.01%
$791	$810	($19)	−2.33%	650 Advertising	$1,890	$7,290	$5,017	68.82%
$106,739	$43,560	$63,179	145.04%	770 Leases & Rentals	$428,035	$392,039	$46,413	11.84%
$945	$485	$460	94.99%	890 Dues & Subscriptions	$4,425	$4,351	$10,491	241.12%
$277	$0	$277	ERR	920 Travel & Education	$7,648	$0	$18,065	0.00%
$315	$1,620	($1,305)	−80.58%	930 Misc Supplies & Expenses	$4,659	$14,580	$496	3.40%
$1,048	$1,350	($302)	−22.40%	950 Freight	$3,837	$12,150	$2,140	17.31%
$377,968	$367,732	$10,236	2.78%	Total Expenses	$3,934,753	$3,521,116	$424,054	8.35%
				Revenue				
$285,858	$329,620	($43,762)	−13.28%	In Patient	$2,570,847	$2,583,866	($13,019)	−0.50%
$747,642	$645,894	$101,748	15.75%	Out Patient	$5,984,473	$5,575,734	$408,740	7.33%
$1,033,501	$975,514	$57,897	2.48%		$8,555,320	$8,159,600	$395,720	6.83%
$655,533	$607,782	$47,751		Margin	$4,620,567	$4,638,484	($28,334)	

Typical monthly variance report.

THE RELATIONSHIP BETWEEN OPERATING COSTS AND PATIENT CHARGES

In the bidding war between provider and payer to establish service prices, there is nothing more important to the survival of a hospital than to keep overhead and operating costs as low as possible. The institution can then hope to balance lower operating costs against lower reimbursement rates. This is in fact the core of all budgeting efforts in all hospitals today. In the past, most hospitals were not adept at translating reduced operating costs into real operations savings because their cost accounting systems were either not in place or not accurate. Hospitals are able to translate operational savings into lower charges for their services or into savings used to reduce the amount of money that would have to be borrowed in the future for new construction or expansion.

MANAGED CARE

Today, managed care organizations are coming on line with increasing force, and reimbursement from these payers is not related to the hospital's overall operating expenses. Instead, the amount of reimbursement is defined during negotiations between the payer and the hospital as provider contracts are negotiated. In many cases, a hospital can either take the deal or leave it. If a hospital takes the deal, its administration must find ways to cut costs and reduce operating expenses so that the amount of reimbursement specified by the contract will more than cover the cost of caring for covered patients. In the current reimbursement environment, establishing charges for services is becoming much less meaningful than it was in the past under the retrospective reimbursement system.

Hospitals require department directors to perform with considerable energy and creativity in order to keep operating costs as low as possible. It is the monthly budget variance report that helps managers track and analyze their financial progress. If departments operate within their budget goals, the probability of the hospital striking contract agreements that are successful with payers increases substantially.

MEASURING THE HOSPITAL'S FINANCIAL CONDITION

After all budget variances are corrected and/or explained, an assessment of the hospital's current financial condition must occur. The organization must maintain a continual process of financial self-evaluation. Due to the frequent passage of new laws and the impact they can have on operations, hospitals must sometimes change course or strategy in midyear. This can only be accomplished effectively if enough reliable information about the facility's fiscal condition is readily at hand. It is the job of the chief financial officer (CFO) not only to have answers in these circumstances, but also to research and keep relevant background data available regarding current trends throughout the industry. The chief financial officer must have the capacity to consider important financial questions in the context of this changing environment and to make recommendations that may have a significant impact on the future direction of the hospital. For example, a hospital may be doing well with respect to the budget and cash flow at midyear. However, because of pending legislation that could impact future revenue, the CFO may recommend changes in current operations. Such a recommendation might be to steer some currently approved expenditures away from a building fund that has been approved in order to increase cash available to cover operating costs. Or conditions may indicate that the institution should increase the percentage of money saved or invested or consider a program or service that the hospital had not considered seriously before. In other instances, approved programs are cancelled.

The overall financial condition of a facility should be measured using three basic measures:

1. Comparison of fiscal performance with other similar facilities around the country and locally
2. Comparison of current fiscal condition against past performance
3. Comparison of the facility's current fiscal condition to its self-stated goals.

Some basic questions hospital administrators must ask at the end of the fiscal cycle are:

1. How much surplus funds do we have over expenses?
2. How does our present condition compare with our budget?
3. From what areas did our surplus in funds come?
4. What are our case mix, payer mix, and collection rates, and what changes in these percentages have we seen from past years' operations?
5. What is the age of our accounts receivable (how promptly is money coming in after billing)?
6. What is our return on equity?
7. What is the return on our investment funds?
8. How do our charges for services compare to those of other similar facilities locally and regionally?
9. What is the institution's cash flow condition (how much cash is readily available for use to cover routine or emergency expenses)?
10. What is our current average net deduction/discounts and what are current trends?
11. What is our debt service (how much interest and principal are we paying on loans, mortgages, and bonds)?

INFORMATION IS POWER AND SURVIVAL

The questions above are fundamental questions to which answers should be readily available. There are tools that can be used by the institution to measure its financial viability as well as how effective it is at carrying out annual budget goals and strategies. You may be at least vaguely aware of such tools as balance sheets and income statements. These are some of the most basic tools CFOs have to evaluate the financial health of their institutions. In addition, there are several financial statements that hospitals use to provide vital financial indicators.

SUMMARY OF COMMON STATEMENTS AND RATIOS FOR MEASURING THE FINANCIAL CONDITION OF A BUSINESS

STATEMENTS
Balance sheet
Income statement
Fund balance
RATIOS
Operating margin
  Measures income, expenses, and revenue over expenses from operations. A high margin indicates high profitability.

Total operating margin
> Shows income, expenses, profit (loss) from operating and nonoperating activity. A high margin indicates high profitability of all incomes—not just operating income.

Days cash on hand
> Measures how much cash or other assets can be quickly liquidated for any given day. Cash flow is very important to an organization. A cash-starved organization is one that cannot move quickly to purchase items or implement programs that may be needed.

Current ratio
> Measures the relationship of all assets and liabilities for a business. Having too high a ratio of liabilities indicates a weak or ailing financial situation.

Total debt ratio
> Shows the relationship between current operating expenses and current and long-term debt. Keeping the amount of total debt in safe relationship with current expenses assures that debt expenses are not getting too great relative to operating expenses.

Debt service as percent of revenue
> Shows the relationship between income and total debt. Helps managers keep current and long-term debt in balance with income or the ability to cover the debt.

Payables index
> Measures the amount of operating expenses in relation to all current liabilities.

Acid test
> Measures cash or funds that can be liquidated quickly with respect to total liabilities.

Growth in fund balance
> Measures how well the various fund balances the hospital has are doing from one period of time to another.

Return on assets
> Measures the amount of assets a business has relative to income to make sure that the assets are in proportion to income. Proper proportion indicates that past income was used wisely.

Although this text does not present a course in financial accounting, it is nevertheless worthwhile for us to appreciate in very general terms the types of tools that hospital managers use to help their institutions meet financial goals. Hospitals prepare annual reports, which are usually made available to interested persons upon request. The annual report contains financial statements listed above as well as others and sometimes offers projections for the coming year. It may also briefly describe some of the specific efforts the institution is making to better serve the community and how plans for future major services will benefit the community. From this financial review, a trained finance person can obtain valuable information in order to gauge the facility's financial strength and ability to make commitments to future programs. We will take a moment to discuss briefly some of the financial statements commonly included in an annual report.

The balance sheet is a statement that defines an organization's current state of wealth. It identifies all the organization's liabilities, assets, and equity. Table 4-3 is the balance sheet of a moderately sized hospital. It is called a balance sheet because of the formula used to construct it: You will note that the amount of money at the bottom of both columns is the same. The balance sheet shows the distribution (relative values or mix) of the hospital's liabilities and assets. A careful review of a balance sheet can provide an indication of a business's financial health and how wisely income has been handled. It indicates, for instance, how much money is committed to long-term debt and the relative amount of cash on hand. The distribution of these monies into assets and liabilities in part indicates how appropriate past financial decisions have been because these past decisions have produced this distribution.

Balance Sheet: Assets = Liabilities + Equities

▶ TABLE 4–3
BALANCE SHEET

ASSETS GENERAL FUNDS			LIABILITIES AND FUND BALANCES	
Current Assets			Current Liabilities	
			Current long term debt	$2,051,881.20
			Accounts payable	$1,277,316.00
Cash and Cash Equivalents	$6,657,392		Accrued salaries, wages & Vacations	$6,451,687
Patient accounts receivable	$22,996,023		Accrued interest payable	$2,088,576
			Anticipated current malpractice costs	$204,179
Inventories	$3,546,314		Other accured expenses	$3,391,689
Prepaid Expenses	$3,934,586			
Other Convertable Assets	$651,836			
			Total Current Liabilities	$15,465,328
Total Current Assets	$37,786,151			
Other limited $ held by board for	$31,257,835		Deferred Rental Income	$231,158
future needs				
Assets needed for specific	$4,046,076		Estimated malpractice costs	$3,147,322
current liabilities				
			Long term debt, excluding installments	$62,431,321
Total Non currnt assets	$27,211,759		Fund balance	$53,827,207
Investments	$6,324,865			
Property, plant and equipment	$62,091,732			
Deferred financing costs	$1,483,288			
Other Assets	$204,540			
Total Assets	$135,102,336		Total liabilities & fund balance	$135,102,335
Donor Restricted Funds			Endowment Funds:	
			Fund Balance	$596,025
Investments	$565,317			

118

INCOME & EXPENSE STATEMENT

Net Patient service revenue	$113,474,191
Other revenue	$2,756,228
Total operating revenue	$116,230,418
Operating Expenses	
Salaries	$54,851,025
Supplies and other expenses	$46,013,831
Depreciation and amortization	$6,620,095
Provision for bad debts	$3,960,785
Interest	$4,369,062
Total Operating Expenses	$115,814,798
Income from operations	$415,620
Nonoperating gains	
Income from investments	$913,444
Income from board designated funds	$290,463
Unrestricted gifts	$343,436
Total nonoperating gains	$1,547,343
Revenue and gains over expenses	$1,962,963
Revenue and gains in excess of expenses	$17,030

COMMONLY USED INDICATORS

Operating margin	0.36%
Total operating margin	1.69%
Payables Index	0.12
Current Ratio	2.44
Return on assets	1.45%
Acid Test	
Growth in fund balance	
Total debt ratio	0.10
Days cash on hand	
Debt service & renenue	

Shows a typical balance sheet and income–expense statement (P&L).

Operating margin provides the results of current business transactions from the perspective of how much money is left after expenses. The accounting tool that is used to show this is the *income and expense statement, statement of profit and loss,* or *statement of revenue and expenses.* It will show gross and net income for a given period of time against expenses for a given period of time, which is usually a month or a quarter. Gross income is the total receipts that were received, and net income is what is left after expenses. A sample of a hospital's income and expense statement can also be seen in Table 4-3. Table 4-4 shows operating margins of hospitals of various sizes.

Income is often referred to in two ways: *operating income* and *nonoperating income.* Operating income is funds received from any aspect of the facility's primary operations. Nonoperating income is income generated independent of normal operations. In the case of hospitals, nonoperating income is primarily gains received from investments. Other types of nonoperating income can come in the form of gifts and donations, but these are sometimes board-designated or limited-funds. Money in these funds is usually allocated by the board or used only as designated by the giver. Funds that are given to a hospital for a specific purpose by the donor are called designated funds and by law must be used only for that stated purpose.

Operating Margin = Current Income − Current Expenses

Growth rate in equity shows growth in fund balances (savings, investments) a business has made. Hospitals generally have several funds, just as one may keep separate savings accounts for various purposes.

It is important to understand that a wide range of factors needs to be sampled before a fa-

▶ TABLE 4−4
HOSPITAL OPERATING MARGINS

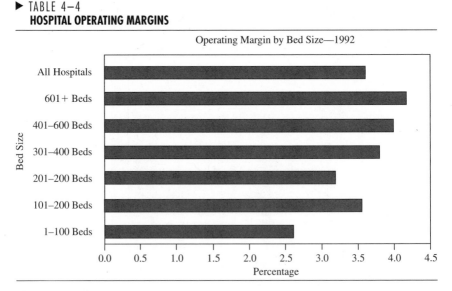

Operating Margin by Bed Size—1992

Shows typical operating margins by size of hospital. Note that, generally, larger hospitals have been able to sustain a slightly higher operating margin than have small hospitals; another example of why mergers are so common today.

(Source: Voluntary Hospitals of America, Inc., Data Comparison Reporting System.)

cility can make a complete fiscal assessment. Hospitals are big businesses, and an 800-bed university facility's annual operating budget can easily exceed $350 million. Such a budget implies enormous complexities resulting from political, operational, and strategic planning efforts. Also, to produce and assess any budge—but particularly a budget of this size—many financial measuring sticks have to be placed carefully throughout the facility's operations. If this is not done, a seemingly obscure element, such as declining available cash on hand, can go unnoticed and lead to more significant difficulties in the future for the institution. For example, declining cash on hand can reflect a gradually increasing account receivables account, and that can result from something going wrong in the billing process. Perhaps coding errors are increasing, resulting in less incoming cash; possibly a quirk in the computer's program has developed. Even more serious implications may result from misunderstood contracts with payers. Table 4-5 shows a typical cash flow statement.

It is also important to understand that various financial monitors have varying degrees of sensitivity. *Sensitivity* in this regard means how quickly these monitors can reflect relatively

---

▶ TABLE 4–5
STATEMENT OF CASH FLOW OF GENERAL FUNDS

Cash flow from operating activities and gains	
Revenue & gains in excess of expenses	$17,030
Adjustments	
Depreciation and amortization	$6,620,095
Provision for bad debts	$3,960,785
Deferred financing costs	$165,992
Increase in pt accounts receivable	($5,248,990)
Increase in inventories	($105,959)
Changes in prepaid expenses	($464,210)
Changes in other assets	$25,223
Changes in accounts payable	($2,130,269)
Increase in accrued salaries and wages benefits	$397,239
Changes in accrued interest payable	($4,932)
Changes in estimated malpractice costs	$1,095,209
Increases in other liabilities	$1,267,361
Net cash from other operations	
Purchases of investments	($153,357)
Proceeds from sales and investments	$61,309,737
Purchases of assets	($62,672,628)
Liquidated funds	$25,253
Purchase of plant and equipment	($7,026,489)
	$0
Net cash used for investments	($851,780)
Cash flow provided by investment activities	
Proceeds from loan funded bonds	($1,002,672)
Net cash provided by financial activities	($1,002,672)
Net increase/decrease in cash and cash equivalent	$4,170,066
Cash and cash equivalent at beginning of year	$8,502,466
Cash and cash equivalent at end of year	$4,332,400

Cash flow indicates the amount of money that is on hand that can be used to pay bills.

subtle changes in operational activity of the facility. It should be pointed out that the financial statements described here are not unique to health care; they are used routinely by for-profit industries as well. In fact, most have been carried into health care from private industry. Also, not all of these statements and ratios are used by all businesses. Many different ratios and statements exist, and the CFO of each facility uses his or her discretion along with board approval as to which of these tools will be used by the organization. Some are used quarterly while others are used monthly or biannually. Others may appears only in annual reports.

STRATEGIC PLANNING: SHORT- AND LONG-RANGE PLANS

To continue providing effective services, a hospital must have a clear idea of its short- and long-range financial goals and also a well-developed strategic plan that will lead to those goals. Planning is often considered in two modes. A short-range plan generally accounts for activities that will occur within two or three years. A long-range plan will consider from 4 to 6 years into the future. Some hospitals engage in even longer-range thinking at times. Because of the dynamic state of the health care industry—not to mention new legislation that can significantly change an organization's entire focus and profitability—five years is about as far as any hospital can seriously project.

People who are typically involved in strategic planning are community leaders, the medical staff, the chief financial officer, key hospital administrators, and the board of directors. Factors that they must consider include current, pending, and proposed legislation and payer groups. In their cost-benefit analysis, they must discuss renovations, new leases, total equipment and building replacement, new technology, plant needs, trash systems, and HVAC (heat, ventilation, and air conditioning).

STRATEGIC PLANNING AND THE EVOLUTION OF PRODUCT LINES

As hospitals and other health care facilities begin to develop their strategic plans in a tight and dynamic economic environment, funds allocated for expansion or new projects must be very seriously considered. Clearly, the mission statement of the institution is again used as a guide. In some instances, it may be necessary to "amend the constitution" and examine how appropriate the facility's current mission statement is under present conditions. Once this evaluation and, if necessary, adjustment is completed, the hospital must then begin to consider which specific plan(s) fit the new mission statement. Clearly, the mission statement must point to services that are affordable as well as in tune with the medical staff's expertise. For instance, a program might be compatible with the mission statement, but the financial resources it requires are not available. Many hospitals have suffered significantly or even closed because too much money was put into carrying out a mission that was too aggressive for the financial condition of the facility.

During the early 1980s, the concept of "product lines" began to evolve more rapidly among health care providers. It is necessary for hospitals to distribute or program their available funds carefully so that only those services that offer a reasonable return on initial investment are funded. In today's market, a reputation for providing excellent service in one or more areas is important because, like good advertising, it helps to generate referrals. It also helps tremendously when negotiating managed care contracts. A hospital must therefore develop a strong reputation for excellence so that payers will want to write contracts for that hospital to take care of the patients they represent. These defined areas of service, if specific enough, become known as products. Such a product might be gene therapy or a center for treating neurological disorders.

CENTERS OF EXCELLENCE AND PRODUCT LINES

Another evolving concept is the establishment of centers of excellence. The establishment of a center of excellence must be supported by an institution's mission statement and appropriate resources. All facilities strive to provide high-quality services. However, a so-called center of excellence is established to provide a "world class" service and to be used as a regional, if not national, center for treatment of a particular disease or disorder. Such a facility can be accomplished only after significant planning and recruitment of prominent physicians, with the support of major capital funding.

Clearly, marketing this service on a regional, national, or even international level is a significant part of the program. These centers operate within the walls of a hospital but are designed to provide a particular service with a very high degree of proficiency. Examples of centers of excellence that might appear in a given hospital are centers for the treatment of neurological, digestive, skeletal, or kidney diseases. Such centers would be recognized as high-level product lines of their institution. It should be pointed out that the facility's basic services would continue, but a significant financial effort would be directed to support these major product lines.

Examples of product lines that may not function at the level of centers of excellence include:

- Organ transplant programs
- Geriatrics centers
- Trauma centers
- Sports medicine centers
- Cancer treatment centers
- Gene therapy centers
- Endocrinology centers

There are many other product lines that can be developed into significant programs. In addition to establishing a high standard of medical care for patients, high-profile product lines provide high public levels of recognition of the overall facility, which in turn can generate additional referrals. Such referrals can involve hospitalization, short-stay surgical procedures, and outpatient testings.

High-profile product lines require substantial resources. Buildings, major equipment purchases, staff, and highly recognized, if not renowned, physicians must be recruited long before the first patient is seen. In fact, the lead time before the first reimbursement payment is received often ranges from 12 to 24 months from the time renovation or construction work begins. This means that facilities must secure loans, or in some instances issue bonds, to fund such programs. In many cases, facilities will budget money for several years in advance from its own operations to fund these programs. Other funding can come from cashing in investments. In many instances not-for-profit hospitals use the money they had been holding.

If the initial assessment of need or the number of referrals associated with such a product line does not meet expectations, it can have a disastrous affect on a hospital's financial status and future growth. Federal laws and changes in payer contracts and agreements can also affect the financial success of these programs. Indeed, these projects involve high-risk–

high-stakes decisions on which the survival of an institution may depend. For example, two large hospitals in an eastern city recently spent many millions of dollars to change their service focuses, one newly focusing on cardiac care, including open-heart surgery, and the second on neurological services. In some instances such major shifts in service are a facility's last chance to stay solvent. These problems give clear evidence why a sound mission statement, good planning, and short as possible construction and implementation schedule become very key elements.

WHO APPROVES THE STRATEGIC PLAN?

The board of directors is ultimately responsible for developing and approving the hospital's short- and long-range strategic plans. However, much of the research and input comes from the hospital's chief financial officer, chief executive officer, and chief operating officer. Like the mission statement, short- and long-range strategic plans are working documents that must be continuously reviewed and revalidated to ensure that they stay compatible with changes in the economy and in legislation. Also, new medical discoveries or new treatment regimens may demand rewriting plans. Such rewriting may include rearranging priorities for programs that have already been approved by the board or adding new services that have not yet been seriously considered. Planners are currently keeping close watch on the evolution of managed care organizations, of capitation contracts, and of new techniques that for the first time allow physicians to perform many procedures on an outpatient basis.

AFFILIATIONS AND NETWORKING AMONG HOSPITALS

In some cases, it is not appropriate for a hospital to launch major new product lines in order to grow or to survive. The alternative may be to affiliate with a much larger or smaller institution. There are several ways such an affiliation can be structured. Figure 4-5 shows the increasing trend toward affiliation and networking. One is an agreement to purchase: hospital A purchases hospital B lock, stock, and barrel. The terms of this purchase/acquisition can vary from cash money to other financial benefits set against operating costs. Such a purchase usually occurs when hospital B is in desperate financial condition and has few alternatives. Figure 4-6 shows organization charts for networking systems.

Rather than an outright purchase, an affiliation may be established between two or more hospitals. In this case, hospital A might be valued by hospital B as an important potential source of new patient referrals: Hospital B may be an active acute care facility that treats many patients but will agree to refer patients who need more complex care to its new affiliate hospital A. Arrangements like this can involve two or several hospitals in an effective network that provides a wide range of services without duplication. Sometimes a large university hospital will develop a network among several small, "feeder" hospitals that will refer patients to the larger hospital, which needs to receive a large number of admissions and to perform a large number of outpatient tests to cover huge overhead and operating expenses.

As part of these affiliation agreements, the smaller hospitals may get an assurance that the larger hospital will help cover some of its operating expenses. Also, the smaller hospital may gain prestige from its association with a university or well-respected tertiary-care facility. Indeed, this new prestige may strengthen all of the facilities within the network by enabling the smaller hospitals to attract more talented physicians.

In some instances, the medical staff of affiliated facilities will participate directly in these

Trends in Hospital Mergers	
Year	Number of Mergers
1985	15
1988	30
1990	13
1994	70

History of Merger and Network Activity

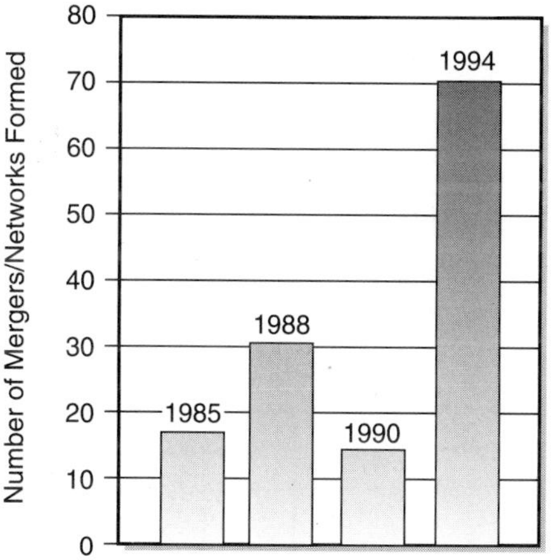

▶ **FIGURE 4-5** Trends toward affiliations and the formation of health care networks (systems) have increased within the last three years. Each of these mergers and networks involves at least two hospitals, and many involve three or four. In some instances, two existing health care systems have merged to become a much larger single system. (Source: The Advisory Board Company, Washington, DC.)

affiliations. In other instances, the medical staff remains within their respective facilities. In the latter case, when patients are moved or referred to another hospital, the receiving hospital's medical staff will take over total treatment of the patient. The patient's initial physicians will receive copies of test reports and other documentation during the patient's visit or upon the patient's return to the original facility. Admitting privileges may be extended to affiliated medical staffs by hospitals within the affiliation.

As in any merger or affiliation, both management and first-line employees feel in jeopardy. In some instances, working relationships and staffing expectations are worked out as part of the final agreement. However, in many instances, the point of the merger or affiliation is to pool resources and to economize where possible. This may mean that some employees will lose their jobs.

More recently, hospitals have begun to purchase individual physician practices. Large family practices and internal medicine practices throughout a given region can generate many referrals to the parent hospital. Today, however, the gain is not to see more patient activity in the facility but rather to encourage HMO payers to write contracts with the hospital. We will see the distinction in the next chapter. Table 4-6 shows the revenue that just a few additional inpatient admissions can yield for a hospital. One of the biggest problems facing hospital administrators today involves maintaining and generating new admissions for those patients who are still on traditional reimbursement contracts. It is equally important for a hospital to gain a healthy mix of admissions because some admission types (DRGs) can yield good incomes while others do not. It is therefore important for an insti-

Fundamental Structure of a Typical Medical Care Delivery Network

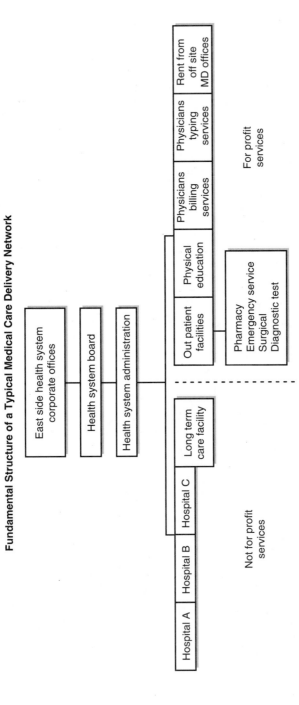

▶ **FIGURE 4–6** A typical networking configuration. There is great variety in how these networks are put together. Some operate with one hospital connected to several outpatient facilities. Other networks/affiliations/mergers may include five or six hospitals in one corporation. The term *network* has also changed recently to include configurations that include payers and providers in one large system. Networking and affiliations provide three important opportunities: group purchasing, reduction of underutilized services (increased efficiency), and stronger leverage when negotiating with managed care payers.

▶ TABLE 4–6
ANNUALIZING GROSS CHARGES FOR INPATIENTS

AVERAGE NUMBER OF ADMISSIONS/YEAR	AVERAGE CHARGE PER ADMISSION	VARIANCE IN CHARGES
18000	$9,000	$162,000,000
18050	$9,000	$162,450,000

NOTE: Net revenue may be in the range of 35% of gross revenue.

Traditionally, in the non-managed-care environment, hospital administrators worked actively to increase the number of admissions. In fact, hospitals spent a great deal of time and money recruiting physicians and developing services that would increase admissions. In many cases, a relatively small number of admissions could have a significant impact on annual revenue. Efforts to bring physicians with special skills on staff as affiliates of a hospital are still going on, but the motive today is that such physicians may give a hospital more negotiating power because these physicians can offer HMO patients better and more comprehensive services at one facility

tution to attract a reasonably balanced ratio of these admissions: It would not help the hospital's bottom line to attract too many low-profit DRGs. Hospitals that purchase practices do so knowing the nature of the admissions that are generated by these practices. Overall, the trend is toward a reduction in patient admissions. There is also constant pressure to reduce length of stay, which reduces operating costs. The combination of these two factors has caused many hospitals to downsize, to permanently close nursing floors to reduce operating cost. In fact in more extreme cases this results in bankruptcy.

Merger, buyout, affiliation, and *networking* are terms that are too often used interchangeably. Sometimes, the net effect of these strategies is similar, but their actual structures can be very different. For example, a health provider system or network can form via a buyout, an affiliation, or a merger.

Today many hospitals need to merge for survival. New initiatives have been forged between entities that had been in almost adversarial relationships. Payers (managed care and others) are joint venturing affiliations with providers (hospitals) and their medical staff to share risk under a provider agreement. Such unions have brought full circle the once very separately motivated interested of payers, hospitals, and physicians into a cost-effective medical delivery system.

Many systems, however, do not involve a buyout. Two or more hospitals may decide that rolling their operations into one corporation requires only an agreement and understanding from both boards, medical staffs, and administrations that joining forces under one system umbrella is mutually beneficial. This understanding and resulting agreements, however, can take up to two years to hammer out. Ultimately, a voluminous and detailed document is filed with the federal government for review and approval. Significant costs accompany the preparation of this document. Several consultants are required to help the medical staff, board, and administration prepare it. Studies of service areas affected, referral patterns, and proposed cost savings to the community are given much scrutiny. Real estate and cash holdings need to be defined along with a description of where and how they will be managed in the future. The price tag for answering these hundreds of complex questions can range from $1 million to $2 million. If the merger is approved, the operations plan for merging all the facilities involved can begin.

(Text continues on page 131)

▲ TABLE 4–7
HOSPITAL UTILIZATION RATES: 1970 TO 1993 (REPRESENTS ESTIMATES OF INPATIENTS DISCHARGED FROM NONINSTITUTIONAL, SHORT-STAY HOSPITALS, EXCLUSIVE OF FEDERAL HOSPITALS. EXCLUDES NEWBORN INFANTS. BASED ON SAMPLE DATA COLLECTED FROM THE NATIONAL HOSPITAL DISCHARGE SURVEY, A SAMPLE SURVEY OF HOSPITAL RECORDS OF PATIENTS DISCHARGED IN YEAR SHOWN; SUBJECT TO SAMPLING VARIABILITY.)

SELECTED CHARACTERISTIC	PATIENTS DISCHARGED (1,000)	PATIENTS DISCHARGED PER 1,000 PERSONS[1]			DAYS OF CARE PER 1,000 PERSONS[1]			AVERAGE STAY (DAYS)		
		Total	Male	Female	Total	Male	Female	Total	Male	Female
1970	29,127	144	118	169	1,122	982	1,251	8.0	8.7	7.6
1980	37,832	168	139	194	1,217	1,068	1,356	7.3	7.7	7.0
1985	35,056	148	124	171	954	849	1,053	6.5	6.9	6.2
1986	34,256	143	121	164	913	817	1,003	6.4	6.8	6.1
1987	33,387	138	116	159	889	806	968	6.4	6.9	6.1
1988[2]	31,146	128	107	147	834	757	907	6.5	7.1	6.2
1989[2]	30,947	126	105	145	815	741	884	6.5	7.0	6.1
1990[2]	30,788	124	102	144	792	704	875	6.4	6.9	6.1
1991[2]	31,098	124	103	144	795	715	869	6.4	7.0	6.0
1992[2]	30,951	122	101	142	751	680	818	6.2	6.7	5.8
1993,[2] total	30,825	120	98	141	720	644	792	6.0	6.5	5.6

Age

Under 1 year old	710	181	206	156	1,155	1,265	1,041	6.4	6.1	6.7
1 to 4 years old	654	41	46	37	163	169	157	3.9	3.7	4.3
5 to 14 years old	777	21	22	20	108	110	105	5.1	5.1	5.2
15 to 24 years old	3,088	87	37	138	309	204	416	3.5	5.5	3.0
25 to 34 years old	4,655	113	53	171	446	313	575	4.0	5.9	3.4
35 to 44 years old	3,457	85	72	99	431	424	438	5.1	5.9	4.4
45 to 64 years old	6,283	127	132	123	785	831	742	6.2	6.3	6.1
65 to 74 years old	4,890	262	284	245	1,927	2,033	1,844	7.4	7.2	7.5
75 years old and over	6,310	446	476	430	3,665	3,764	3,609	8.2	7.9	8.4

Region

Northeast	6,965	136	119	152	952	876	1,023	7.0	7.4	6.7
Midwest	7,097	116	98	134	706	638	771	6.1	6.5	5.8
South	11,580	131	104	156	749	658	834	5.7	6.3	5.4
West	5,183	93	72	114	473	419	527	5.1	5.8	4.6

[1]Based on Bureau of the Census estimated civilian population as of July 1. Estimates for 1980–90 do not reflect revisions based on the 1990 Census of Population. [2]Comparisons beginning 1988 with data for earlier years should be made with caution as estimates of change may reflect improvements in the design rather than true changes in hospital use. (Source: U.S. National Center for Health Statistics, *Vital and Health Statistics*, series 13; and unpublished data.)

Show trends of per capita admissions. Note, the amount of out patient activity relative to the number of admissions. Source, The American Hospital Association.

▶ TABLE 4–8
EIGHT MAJOR CATEGORIES OF NETWORK SAVING

	TRADITIONAL NETWORK COST SAVING STRATEGIES					RADICAL STRATEGIES		INFRASTRUCTURE STRATEGY
I Renegotiating Contracts	**II** Consolidating Management	**III** Consolidating Support Function	**IV** Merging Sub-Scale Clinical Un	**V** Segregating Complex and Routine Procedures	**VI** Closing Subscale Hospitals	**VII** Creating a Sheel "Hospital"	**VIII** Creating the Intelligent Network
Networks eliminate duplicate contracts and use volume-based leverage to win favorable terms for supply and service contracts, loans, and insurance.	Systems centralized management functions and administrative departments, eliminate duplicative positions.	Networks centralize entire operational and clinical support departments (e.g., laboratory, laundry, finance). Do not require proximity to care delivery site.	Networks close under-utilized clinical units and transfer patient volume to other network facilities.	Networks triage complex cases to a designated specialty center leaving routine cases in other system hospitals.	Systems close hospital(s) and transfer patients to other network facilities.	Systems remove acute care services from low-occupancy hospitals and re-orient them to nonacute care.	System invests in highly capable central network administrative staff who are able to chart strategic vision for group. Identify and disseminate "best practices" for adoption across system.
Advisory Grade A	A	A–	C	B	A/C, 2	C	A
Potential Savings As a % of Total Hospital Cost 3.0%	4.5%	3.1%	0.8%	1.3%			

A = Tactic recommended for virtually all networks; large potential cost savings and low risk of revenue loss

C = Tactic worthy of serious consideration by all networks; moderate savings potential and manageable risk of revenue loss

C = Tactic not worth pursuing for most networks

1 = Tactic has been assigned two grades, as assessment of idea will vary depending on circumstances. Closure is an "A" idea for networks with facilities in close proximity to each other, but a "C" idea for networks in which all hospitals serve distinct communities, physician groups.

2 = Estimates for a five hospital system. Calculation possible only for traditional cost savings strategies. Large dollars available as well from full closure of hospital; actual net savings turn on number of hospitals closed and percentage of patient revenues retained by system.

Outlines cost savings and new revenue opportunities that occur through mergers and networking.

Sometimes these "applications to merge" are not approved by the federal government. For example, the government may feel that if the merger of two or more hospitals occurs, those facilities will be in a much stronger position to control and define how health care is to be provided in their joint service area. In other words, the government may view the merger as offering too strong a possibility of restraint of trade: Such a merger might work against the likelihood of other health care providers who want to set up shop in the area, leading to lack of competition that could give the merged facilities too much control over service charges in their area. Also a lack of competition may affect quality and scope of services provided to the community

Affiliations tend to be less complex and threatening to restraint of trade statutes because they depend on each facility operating generally as it has done in the past, although each facility may have specific responsibility to provide key services under certain conditions that are defined by the affiliation agreement. There is no formal merging or changes in ownership, and the resulting documentation is much less complex.

OTHER CONSIDERATIONS THAT AFFECT A STRATEGIC PLAN

Community needs must be high on the list of considerations in any hospital strategic plan. A requirement of all not-for-profit hospitals is to function as the custodian of the community's health resources. For this reason, hospital administrators continuously keep in touch with the community through contact with professional groups, business organizations (such as local merchants' organizations), and service organizations (such as the Lions Club and the Rotary Club). These are just a few sources that provide hospital administrators and board members with impressions of community health care needs.

The medical staff can also have a profound effect on the development of the strategic plan. We saw earlier that hospitals are beginning to position themselves through active advertising so that they can provide more specific or expanded product lines. Many large university-based hospitals are developing very expensive gene research programs that will probably lead to future clinical applications. Clearly, programs that involve new or expanded product lines such as this are not possible without a prominent medical director and huge financial resources. In many cases, new product lines may be substantial enough to support other basic hospital services that are necessary but unprofitable.

On the other side of the coin, however, are hospital strategic plans that have ended in financial chaos when a well-recognized physician or group of physicians leaves an institution without warning. Hospitals frequently conduct secret bidding wars over prominent physicians and physician groups. Hospitals that lose physicians in these battles may also lose a significant number of referrals, or in some circumstances, the entire service a physician was involved in.

The general characteristics or personality of the medical staff also affect an organization's planning. The author has observed different hospitals whose medical staffs viewed working with new medical techniques very differently. For instance, one staff felt positively challenged through peer pressure to write papers about a new technique and to extend themselves to teach as guest lecturers at university-based hospitals. In the same town, the staff at another hospital was not nearly as aggressive in adopting the new technique. Clearly, the strategic plans for these two facilities would have to be compatible with the characteristics of their staffs. The short- and long-range goals for these facilities would also be very different.

The federal government can certainly influence the strategic plan through legislation that can ultimately create new trends in medical care. Also, it can impose limitations on new programs a hospital may want to consider. The certificate of need (CON) laws, for example, which were once present in every state, simply prevented a hospital from installing equipment, instituting new programs, or building a new structure if, under CON criteria, the new effort "did not meet or exceeded community needs." CON regulations are the residual of tight institutional control by the federal government under the 1964 Medicare plan. Some states continued the program but altered the criteria significantly. Some others did not. Government regulations on health care providers can cause havoc as easily as they can provide benefits to the health care delivery system.

IMPLEMENTATION OF A PRODUCT LINE AND THE FEASIBILITY STUDY

Each new or expanded product line or program must be rolled into the operating and capital budgets for final board approval before it can be put into motion. Comprehensive business plans must be prepared and a detailed evaluation of the program conducted. In many cases, the first step toward approving a product line is to fund a feasibility study. Feasibility studies can take up to 12 months to complete, depending on the complexity of the program. Most often, these studies are researched and prepared by outside consultants who have been hired by the hospital with board-approved funds. Once this step has been completed, the program can be approved by the hospital and budgeted.

The feasibility study will identify such key elements as:

- Demand for the proposed service
- Cost of project
- Building renovation costs
- Operating costs
  - Indirect costs
  - Direct operating costs
- Capital costs
- Impact on institution if program is not implemented

More detailed cost and revenue projections must then be included in the facility's final budget. It is necessary to show the financial, administrative, and service matters the project is expected to address. An example of a business plan for a small project will be discussed in more detail later in a discussion regarding the radiology budget and will contain the essential elements of a comprehensive feasibility plan. Suffice it to say now that a typical business plan for, say, a $10 million project could easily run to 100 pages. As noted earlier, embarking on such large projects is done these days only with great caution.

STUDY QUESTIONS

1. Approximately what percentage of overall health care expenses is attributed to hospital service?
2. If you were an administrator, how would you explain the need for implementing a strong budget variance reporting policy? How would you define a budget and the value it has to an organization?
3. What considerations are essential to keep in mind when developing a mission statement? What group(s) of people would you solicit for help in the task and why?

4. Explain the following. You may use examples to explain.

   Operating budget
   Capital budget
   Direct expenses
   Variable expenses
   Depreciation expense

5. Explain the responsibilities each of the positions below has in developing a budget.

   Board of directors
   Chief operating officer
   Chief financial officer
   Vice president of services
   Department director
   Department chairperson

6. If you were the chief executive officer of a hospital and felt a need to develop a new product line, what should you consider before presenting your ideas to the board of directors for initial discussion? If the board feels positive about the new program, what is your next step?

7. Why is it important to understand as much as possible about what type of legislation the state or federal government is planning?

8. What characteristics and capabilities would you look for in a chief financial officer for your hospital?

9. Briefly explain why the following factors affect budget variances, and give an example for each factor.

   Inventory
   Internal purchase order processing procedures
   Negotiating package deals with vendors
   Short lead time delivery of supplies

10. As a CFO, what statements and information would you want to present to the board during a regularly scheduled meeting to keep them up-to-date about the hospital's financial condition?

11. Briefly explain how changes in the following can affect a hospital's financial picture.

    Length of stay
    Number of admissions per year
    Occupancy
    Acuity index
    Payer mix
    Average length of accounts receivable

12. If you were part of a negotiating group that is working with an HMO to settle a multiyear contract, how would you go about understanding the value of, and agreeing to, a given discount off "list" that they are proposing?

13. Explain the following:

    Operating margin
    Cash flow
    Credit ratio
    Debt to service ratio
    Profit and loss

14. What does the balance sheet tell you about an organization's financial condition? What is the formula for developing a balance sheet?

15. What does the P&L statement show? What is the formula for developing this statement?

16. What is overhead? Give two examples.

17. What groups of people would you gather to help you develop a five-year strategic plan for your hospital? Give examples of three new product lines you might want to recommend for consideration and their possible benefit to the organization and to the community. Keep in mind specific circumstances that would make you consider expanding services as opposed to cutting services to reduce expenses.

18. Imagine that you are the chief administrative officer of a 350-bed hospital that struggled to break even last year. You are approached by a large tertiary-care facility and asked to consider a buyout or an affiliation. What factors would be important to consider? What factors would the medical staff be concerned about? Would you prefer a buyout or an affiliation?

19. Write at least a half-page summary that explains the capital budget by addressing the following:

    What expenses it covers
    The role of the board and hospital administrators
    The role of the medical staff
    The role of the community

20. Explain depreciation, and give a brief example by calculating straight line depreciation expenses for a piece of equipment that was purchased at a cost of $200,000 and has a life expectancy of eight years. Also explain which budget would carry these expenses.

21. As a department director, you receive a budget variance for two line items that are outside accepted limits. One is for medical surgical supplies (which includes syringes, catheters, tubing, etc.), and the other is for X-ray equipment repair services. What steps would you take to understand these variances?

FIVE

The Health Care Insurance System

OBJECTIVES FOR STUDY

After reading this chapter, the student will

▶ Appreciate the services that other major industrial countries offer as parts of their national health care programs.

▶ Appreciate the fundamental advantages and disadvantages of a national health care system.

▶ Appreciate the fundamentals of how federal and state governments influence health care expenses and what portion of the overall health care bill they actually pay.

▶ Appreciate the conflicts that will occur as the current demand for high-quality health care remains in force, the availability of services is extended to more of the population, yet available financial resources decline.

▶ Understand how legislation affects the payment structure and operating policies of a hospital.

▶ Appreciate the two philosophies regarding future government involvement in the funding and control of health care services.

▶ Appreciate the effect that rising health care costs have on a nation's economy and why the gross national product (GNP) is used to measure economic inflation in the health care industry.

▶ Understand the fundamentals of payer mix, discounting, and the collection rate and why hospitals need to be concerned about these factors.

▶ Appreciate the basic issues regarding hospitals' engagement in contract services with HMOs and PPOs.

▸ Understand the reasons behind the growing popularity of health care maintenance organizations.

▸ Appreciate the basic structures of HMOs and PPOs and their effect on overall health care costs.

▸ Understand the basic meaning of the following terms: *patient days, per diem, length of stay, managed care.*

WHO PAYS THE BILL?

In the United States, the answer to this question has usually been either third-party payers or the government—not the patient. A third-party payer is an insurance company (carrier) who pays a health care provider on behalf of a group plan or individual policy holder. This system is unlike those in other advanced industrial countries, where governments, not commercial insurers, pay nearly all health care bills. Until the Social Security Act, which established the Medicare and Medicaid programs, was signed into law in 1964, there has been two primary insurer groups in the United States. The first was the Blue Cross and Blue Shield system, which covered most of the population by far. It provided both group and individual policies either directly to individuals or through employee group plans. The Blues, as they are sometimes called, are nonprofit organizations, and their plans had been called indemnity policies. The second group of insurers is made up of private for-profit insurance companies, such as Aetna, Metropolitan, and the Prudential.

In the United States today, most health insurance subscribers are covered through premiums that are part of their employers' benefit packages. Figure 5-1 shows the distribution of payers of health care costs generated by hospitals in the United States. Although the author will not attempt to describe here the multitude of health insurance plans available, the

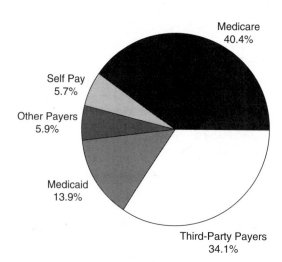

Community Hospital Gross Patient Revenue by Payer Source, 1992

Medicare 40.4%

Self Pay 5.7%

Other Payers 5.9%

Medicaid 13.9%

Third-Party Payers 34.1%

▸ **FIGURE 5–1** Shows the distribution of payers of costs generated by community hospitals. This distribution is expected to change dramatically as managed care organizations enter the mix, which is already occurring rapidly in the East and the South. (Source: The American Hospital Association.)

reader should be aware that there are enough options and variations among these policies that many employers keep consultants available to provide information to their employees regarding the scope and details of the benefits offered through the various companies.

BRIEF OVERVIEW OF NATIONAL HEALTH PLANS AROUND THE WORLD

In most other industrialized countries, health care costs are covered under national plans. Under most such plans, most health care facilities are in effect owned and operated by the national government. The government sets rules regarding the type, scope, and limitations of and exceptions to the coverage that its citizens will receive. There are usually some private commercial health care facilities that operate independent of the national government which provide patient services as a supplement to the national plan. In other words, many people who have the means to pay extra premiums subscribe to these companies for additional coverage. Those who cannot afford the price of private supplemental insurance must rely exclusively on the national health plan.

Since the government owns and buys almost all the equipment under many of these national health plans, many health care workers including physicians are government employees. The government can regulate the number of pieces of equipment that will be used throughout the country simply by controlling the capitated rate or budget. Here to, certain patients may not have open access to equipment for a test that is medically indicated. The author has experienced through discussions with a close relative who lived in one of the more advanced countries with a national medical plan. This personal experience provided insights that are not so apparent from the outside. This personal experience saw a middle-aged person refused priority heart catheterization, and hospitalization because of long waiting times by other people. The delays in testing and treatment she experienced would not be imagined in the U.S. today, yet it was not uncommon in this country. The result of this is that if she had not accepted experimental surgery she would had not survived the delays that were built into their health care system.

Although this is one specific event, it clearly points out that nationalized health care and capitated rates of any kind does not come without the potential of serious limitations to patient access for services. Extremes at either end of the service are certainly not appropriate, and surely the United States health care delivery system may be accused of operating on the side of excess in some areas. Our current efforts to investigate and design a national health plan that will fit the needs of our culture and the nation's pocket book will continue to be debated and re-evaluated for some into the future.

Only the United States and South Africa do not have comprehensive national health care plans. However, the United States does have Medicare and Medicaid which in many ways qualiifies as this type of coverage.

In 1883, Germany became the first country to start multitrade access to a social health care insurance plan. The plan covered workers in factories, mines, and other trades. Sweden, Hungary, and Australia soon followed suit. The United Kingdom launched the British National Health Service in 1911.

The Canadian health care system has been seen as a potential model by the United States as it considers moving toward a national health care program. The reason for this lies in part in the relative similarities between the two countries in terms of overall lifestyle, economics, and location and in the perceived success of the Canadian system. Under the Canadian system, each province receives a capitated (per capita) amount of money each year which is distributed to its various hospitals. Each hospital is then required to provide all needed services to its population with that amount. Funding is decided each year by the national government. Private health care insurance has been almost entirely eliminated, although it does exist for those who can pay out-of-pocket premiums.

Like other countries, Canada can claim universal coverage for its citizens; however, it may not be able to claim that its citizens have access to medical services to the degree that many in the United States have under current coverage. The fundamental reason for this may in part lie in Canada's having a much lower rate of inflation of medical spending than does the United States. Over the last 20 years, Canada's health care spending measured against its GNP has increased by approximately 3.5%, as compared to an increase of almost 8% in the U.S. New technology seems to become available for widespread use across the country more slowly in Canada than in the United States, and, as noted above, this can translate into limited access by current U.S. standards.

The long wait for diagnostic testing and delays for hospital admissions and surgical procedures common in Canada may not be tolerated in the United States. Yet the U.S. system has encouraged significant waste of resources, which has driven intolerable increases in health care costs. These increases in expenses have not yielded equally significant increases in the U.S. population's state of overall healthfulness, which compares poorly to some countries that have more limited-access health care programs. U.S. mortality and morbidity rates, for example, are actually higher than those of some other developed nations. The answer to the question of how to measure the effectiveness of medical care, however, is still illusive. Important questions remain concerning how to determine the appropriate number of health care units and services that should be available.

Germany's medical system is paid for by "sickness funds," which are managed by nonprofit organizations that are sanctioned by the government to collect premiums through payroll deductions. These organizations act as an administration and distribution service that works for the government. Each citizen must enroll with a sickness fund organization, and those who are unemployed have their premiums covered by the government. Phelps reports that the average premium amounts to approximately 13% of an employee's wages. Physicians in Germany are paid from the sickness funds; however, these funds are distributed first to a physician's association. The physician then receives income based on the contractual agreement with the physician's association.

Japan's health care program consists of a large number of private not-for-profit hospitals and an additional group of government hospitals. Health care coverage, as in Germany, is mandatory for all citizens. Japan reports the lowest number of hospital admissions per capita in the world—approximately 5.7 per 100 people. The United States, Canada, and the United Kingdom experience twice that amount. This is in part attributable to Japan's strong dependence on ambulatory care, which occurs through doctors' visits to patients' homes and a well-developed system of outpatient clinics. Japan's relatively low-cost medical care program yields relatively effective outcomes. Life expectancies for both men and women are slightly higher and infant mortality rates slightly lower than in many industrialized countries. Lifestyle and diet in Japan—not the medical system per se—may have an important impact, along with the average age of the country's population on these statistics. Figure 5-2 shows the percentage of various countries' GNPs that is given to health care. Table 5-1 shows how these comparisons relate to per capita costs.

In all of these systems, a more or less acceptable balance of costs and services has been achieved, which is based on expectations that are part of each country's history and culture. The United States population tends to place access to advanced services and availability of a wide scope of services higher on its scale of expectations than do the populations of other countries.

Our challenge in health care today is to define the value of our health care services to a

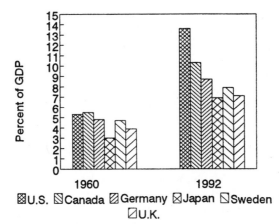

▶ **FIGURE 5-2** Illustrates the growth of medical expenses relative to various countries' GNPs during a period of rapid growth in all health care systems. (Source: U.S. Health and Human Services.)

degree that has not been required in the past. Congressional disputes concerning health care access and coverage appear at least on the surface too motivated by political considerations to produce an intelligent national health care program for the people Congress represents. However, these disputes have also been the result of Congress members studying the U.S. health care system to a level of detail previously unseen, which in turn has resulted in a realization that there is indeed no free lunch at the health care table. With this lesson firmly fixed in the minds of both the general population and its political representatives, cuts in cost had to be found. Such cuts seriously threaten the incomes of large provider groups, such as hospitals and physicians.

How much should this country pay for health care and how much access should individuals have to services are central questions in these disputes. Access has two components. The first involves whether—and by whom—the costs of services for an individual will be paid. The second involves whether or not those services are available when needed. Very few industrialized countries have both components fully in place because this is very expensive to accomplish. The degree to which these disputes are eventually resolved will be determined by the level of creativity and concern for quality of services shown by repre-

▶ TABLE 5-1
RELATIVE HEALTH CARE EXPENDITURES WITH OTHER INDUSTRIAL COUNTRIES

	PERCENT OF GDP		AVERAGE COST FOR HEALTH CARE PER CAPITA
	1980	1992	1992
Canada	7%	13.6%	$1,949
Germany	8.6%	8.7%	$1,775
Japan	6.8%	6.9%	$1,376
United States	9.1%	13.6%	$3,086

Source: National Center for Health Statistics, Public Health Services.

Shows comparative health care expenditures and per capita annual costs.

sentatives in Washington. In fact, the private sector has shown significant progress through the growing acceptance of the managed care approach. Similarly, both hospitals and physicians are beginning to make adjustments in order to cope with this evolution of non-government health care reform.

NATIONAL HEALTH CARE PROGRAMS IN THE UNITED STATES

The United States implemented its first social health care program for the mentally ill in the late 1800s. In 1878, the United States created the Marine Hospital Service, which became the first U.S. government-organized health service plan. Its initial aim was to cover merchant sailors, but this later broadened to include miners and selected other workers whose trades were considered vital to the country's growth. In the early 1900s, the American Association for Labor Legislation organization was formed to advocate social health care programs. There was great skepticism among people about the government establishing these plans, and hospital administrators and physicians questioned the appropriateness of government involvement. But gradually, government intervention was supported by the newly formed American Hospital Association. As the Great Depression gripped the country, a group called the Committee on the Cost of Medical Care was formed and advocated that large sums of tax money be used to cover the growing health care costs of those who could not pay. Another significant movement toward social insurance legislation occurred in the early 1930s and resulted in the Social Security Program of 1935.

The New Deal did not include public money to cover health care programs, however. President Roosevelt strongly advocated the National Health Conference as a form of social health care insurance but this was defeated by Congress. President Truman also lobbied for a social health care plan, but the concept once again failed. The overriding public belief was that government and health care should not mix. Some people were concerned about rapidly rising costs that would lead to increased taxes. Others believed that the government would be too cumbersome and aloof to make the right changes in the system.

Despite these concerns, advances in medical techniques began to evolve rapidly after World War II. As these advances continued, more and more physicians and nurses trained for service. Also, as the benefits of such advances became more apparent to the general public, the demand for health care services rocketed, which in turn led to a rapid widening of the scope of available services that occurred throughout the 1940s, 1950s, and 1960s. However, only a relatively small number of people were covered by health insurance of any type: In 1945, for instance, only about 32 million people had any degree of insurance coverage. Still, pressure continued to build for access to health care services, and this ultimately encouraged the federal government to develop and implement legislation that would cover the cost of health care services provided to the disadvantaged, particularly the elderly and those living at or below the poverty level. This trend toward entitlement led to the 1964 Social Security Act, which created the Medicare and Medicaid programs.

MEDICARE PROGRAMS

The projected cost of the Medicare program was enormous, and funds were to be taken from the cash reserves in the Social Security coffers, from contributions made by employee-employer personnel benefit packages, and from new taxes. Approximately 75% of the funds that were needed to support the program came from federal government sources and the rest from employee-employer contributions. Under this act, Part A and Part B

Medicare Plans were developed. Part A provided compulsory coverage for all persons age 65 or over for *inpatient* hospital services. Part B paid for a percentage of the physician's list price. The list price is established by physicians but must be considered "reasonable" by Medicare administrators. Even so, there are gaps in Medicare coverage, and many people age 65 or over have to pay to fill these gaps. Supplemental insurance designed to close these gaps in coverage is available to individuals through private insurance companies. In 1991, Medicare beneficiaries were liable for, on average, approximately 23% of their total hospital bills.

Approximately 40 million people were not covered in 1995 by any form of health care insurance. This problem began to receive considerable attention in the early 1990s and became one of the central issues in the 1992 presidential elections because Bill Clinton campaigned in part on a promise to drastically reduce this number.

MEDICAID: THE STATE GOVERNMENT HEALTH PLAN

The 1964 Social Security legislation also mandated that federal funds be distributed to each state to care for the nation's indigent population. The principal criterion for eligibility was and is the patient's or family's annual income. These funds were to be combined with funds provided by each state to create a pool of money to be used to support the Medicaid program. In effect, each state was given a charter to administer its own Medicaid program under general federal guidelines. Each state had to find ways to generate its portion of funding, which in many instances resulted in increased state income taxes. Other state funding came from funds redistributed from the state's other services and programs. Federal funds flowing to the states were calculated on a per capita basis: In other words, the more people living in a state, the more funding came from the federal government. Because each state administered its program differently, state Medicaid payment and coverage plans varied considerably.

When the Medicaid plan was initially developed, federal funds covered approximately 83% of each state's costs but in 1995 federal funding dropped to approximately 75%.

Although the Medicare and Medicaid programs are certainly a form of socialized health care programs, the United States generally does not view itself as having a nationalized health plan. There are several contributing factors as to why the United States did not follow the lead of the European countries.

- The United States is a much more heterogeneous society.
- Americans have been very vocal and more effective in expressing their distrust of programs that are fully controlled by the government.
- A more highly developed and comprehensive network of private insurance companies came into being faster than government programs could be developed.
- The age of the population was relatively young.
- Employers were willing to provide insurance through private carriers for their employees.
- Employers, rather than the government, moved to develop early programs, which established a pattern of employer-linked insurance.

FINDING WAYS TO REDUCE INSURANCE PREMIUMS

When the cost of health care rises relative to the GNP, there is great pressure to reduce and control costs. To reduce their costs, payers are scrutinizing the charges they receive from providers. Insurance premiums almost always reflect not only direct costs for services that patients receive, but also other operating costs that are averaged into each charge. In other words, "cost loading" occurs. The price of an automobile, for example, includes more than just the cost of the worker hours of assembly time and the materials needed to produce the car. Advertising costs, employee training expenses, utility bills, the cost of employee pension plans, and more are all rolled into the selling price. In addition to these costs, a percentage is added for profit. Without this profit percentage, there would be little incentive to provide any product or service.

The same is true with hospitals. However, people do not usually pay directly for hospital services; an insurance company or government pays most of the bill. As we know, in the past, under the retrospective payment system, the amount of money paid to the provider for inpatient services was dependent on the expenses generated by the provider. Today, reimbursement is more often paid up front for inpatient services, and the amount paid to hospitals is precalculated and based on the disease category, or DRG. (As you will remember, this is called prospective payment.) This was obviously a major change that concerned all providers. As pressure continued to bring the cost of health care down further, managed care organizations (HMOs) became more popular. These organizations also use the prospective payment model. Once an HMO signs subscribers, which can number into the hundreds of thousands, it will approach a provider to negotiate a contract for services. This contract generally requires that the HMO's subscribers will be sent only to the providers designated in the contract. The contract payment rate is sometimes based on per visit charges, but recently this rate is more often simply a fixed annual fee. We refer to the former as a fee-for-service contract and the latter as a capitated or capped contract.

Not all patients who receive care in a hospital are associated with HMO plans. In fact, some are still covered by payers who reimburse based on a percentage of the list price of the service, although the number of these payers is declining rapidly.

HMO CONTRACT NEGOTIATIONS

An HMO may come to a hospital or freestanding facility to negotiate a blanket charge for providing health care services to its subscribers. The HMO contract is appealing to hospitals because of the large number of patients and the guaranteed revenue it can potentially bring to the hospital. However, in return for that contract, the HMO will want the hospital to agree to healthy discounts if reimbursement is based on the fee-for-service model. If the contract is a capitated agreement, the HMO will want to negotiate the lowest possible annual fee to cover all health care services for its subscribers.

Under the fee-for-service model, a heavily discounted agreement might be worthwhile for the hospital if it insures a high volume of patients. Under a capitated plan, on the other hand, the hospital is hoping patient volume to be very low because each patient who receives services under the capitated contract takes away from the facility's potential profits or guaranteed income. Hospitals have been racheting down costs during the last few years, and there is a serious question now as to how much more discounting can occur before the availability of services and quality are seriously affected. We stated earlier that the single most important question in health care today is how to find the balance point between low cost and high quality of service. This process of racheting down costs with tougher payer-provider agreements represents the first significant step toward answering that question.

The U.S. health care system has been criticized severely for its lack of universal coverage. But we must also recognize that the quality and availability of health care services that the vast majority of citizens does receive is unmatched elsewhere in the world. This is both good and bad news. The reality is that nationalized health care systems in other countries provide certain services to all patients at no out-of-pocket cost, but in many instances the scope of these services is limited. Such limited availability would not be tolerated by most Americans today.

PAYER MIX AND COLLECTION RATES

Except for patients who receive health care services under capitated contracts, the amount of net revenue a hospital receives is based on payer mix and collection rates. For example, providers usually receive patients covered by a wide variety of payers, including Medicare, Medicaid, commercial insurance companies, Blue Cross, and HMOs. The distribution of payers for a particular provider is known as the payer mix.

It is likely that different payers will be working with the provider under agreements that have different payment rates. One agreement will have reimbursement set at 50% of list price, while another will be set at 40% or 60%. So if a patient covered by the first payer receives a diagnostic test that has a "list" charge of $120, the provider might actually receive only $60 for performing the test; it may receive more or less from other payers. The actual amount received is referred to as the collection. Collection rate (the percentage of what is actually received from list price) averages 70%. One can more clearly see what happens to a hospital's net income when we look at an entire department (Table 5-2). Clearly, the combination of payer mix and collection rate will have a profound effect on whether a hospital will be able to afford a new program or new technology or even to continue to operate.

In some instances, as we saw in Table 5-1, the collection rate is extremely low. Clearly, if net income is not sufficient to cover the above costs and other legitimate expenses, the facility cannot provide future services.

THE EFFECT INSURANCE COMPANIES HAVE ON HEALTH CARE COSTS

Continuous collaboration between the provider, insurer, and patient aimed at striking an optimal combination of cost and quality of services is necessary to keep down insurance premiums. In the past, under fee-for-service agreements, we have seen the irony that the availability of a third party to pay for services will actually encourage demand for those services. Not having to deal directly with the cost, most patients were not opposed to having medications prescribed, to being referred to specialists, or to having a high number of diagnostic tests performed. This was especially true when their insurance premium payments were covered in total or to a great extent by their employers. This system also tended to insulate physicians from the consequences of increasing their patients' out-of-pocket expenses when ordering tests and recommending treatment plans. Clearly, an alternative system needed to be defined and implemented. Five fundamental building blocks of an economically sound and effective health care system are:

- An optimal number of health care resources
- An optimal mix of resources
- An optimal distribution of resources
- An optimal allocation of resources between current, education, and research programs
- Appropriate supervision of the development and application of technology

▶ TABLE 5–2
ANNUAL VOLUME AND REIMBURSEMENT CALCULATIONS FOR A HYPOTHETICAL FREESTANDING FACILITY

| | Volume by Exam | Cost per Exam | Gross Charges | MEDICARE | | BLUE CROSS | | HMO/A | | HMO/B | | OTHER PAYERS | | Net Reim-bursement |
				Payer Mix	Collec-tion	Payer Mix	Collec-tion	Payer Mix	Collec-tion	Payer Mix	Collec-tion	Payer Mix	Collec-tion	
Ultrasound	3700	$159	$588,300	50%	35%	20%	38%	12%	33%	13%	60%	5%	70%	$240,968
Chest/ribs	5000	$57	$285,000	50%	35%	20%	38%	12%	33%	13%	60%	5%	70%	$116,736
HIP/ABD/pelvis	1200	$267	$320,400	50%	35%	20%	38%	12%	33%	13%	60%	5%	70%	$131,236
Spine	900	$75	$67,500	50%	35%	20%	38%	12%	33%	13%	60%	5%	70%	$27,648
Mammo	10000	$86	$860,000	50%	35%	20%	38%	12%	33%	13%	60%	5%	70%	$352,256
Distal extrem	2500	$57	$142,500	50%	35%	20%	38%	12%	33%	13%	60%	5%	70%	$58,368
Head	1200	$75	$90,000	50%	35%	20%	38%	12%	33%	13%	60%	5%	70%	$36,864
Total	24500		$2,353,700	50%	35%	20%	38%	12%	33%	13%	60%	5%	70%	$964,076

Demonstrates how both payer mix and collection rate affects net income. Note the significant difference between total charges and net income. Also, remember that in most instances today, charges to inpatients have little or no meaning because hospitals are reimbursed by DRG up front rather than by costs for services provided.

MANAGED HEALTH CARE ORGANIZATIONS

(HMOs)

A new way of providing health care coverage was offered to a group of employers in California in 1942. This approach was revolutionary because the same organization provided both the service and the payment. The Kaiser-Permanente company developed a program that was very similar to what we know today as managed health care, or, in other words, a health maintenance organization (HMO). Under the purest HMO model, provider and payer are one in the same. There are many organizational variations from one HMO to another; however, the one prevailing concept is that physicians and providers are in a fairly direct fashion managed by the payer. In the Kaiser-Permanente system, the HMO owned and operated hospitals and outpatient facilities, employing physicians on a salary basis. To form this organization, the company used all the money it would have paid hospitals, physicians, and other providers and built hospitals and hired physicians: instead of Kaiser-Permanente paying premiums to insurance companies for its employees' health care expenses, it used the money to operate its own health care provider service. In doing so, it was able build its own medical staff which could set rules to help monitor the appropriateness of tests, treatments, and other services. These controls are a cornerstone of the system encouraging the overall cost effectiveness that has been a hallmark of HMOs. In some instances, when necessary equipment or expertise is not present in the HMO, patients are sent to outside, private physicians. The HMO concept is thus in some ways analogous to some countries' national health programs.

As noted above, there are several variations in how HMOs are organized. The Kaiser-Permanente plan is the purest form in that it owns and controls almost all aspects of the program. Other HMOs employ no physicians but instead write contracts with private physician groups to treat their HMO patients on a fee-for-service basis or for a capitated annual fee. All patients in such HMOs must see only those physicians and facilities identified in such agreements. HMOs will also write contracts with other providers, such as hospitals and other freestanding facilities.

HMOs have leverage to negotiate discounts because they will approach more than one provider. This creates "managed competition," as bidding or negotiations among providers drives the discount. Hospitals and other providers in exchange look for exclusivity. As part of the negotiating process with the provider, an HMO will try to package an agreement that includes the largest possible pool of subscribers. In this way, the provider gets a sufficient number of patients to make the discounting worthwhile. In other words, hospitals will accept contracts that show lower income per exam if it is based on a large number of lives under capitated contract as shown in Table 3-1.

In order for hospitals to negotiate intelligently with HMOs, they must have a clear understanding of their operating costs. If operating costs are not known, the provider will not be able to negotiate successfully with a payer. If these costs are known, the hospital can create a model that estimates patient activity and expenses that will be incurred for providing services to these patients. The model will also show the net income the provider can expect from the deal. For example, providers can use a growing data base that shows how many diagnostic tests, admissions, births, and so on can be expected for a population of 100,000. This population can also be subdivided into characteristic utilization rates. A population that has an average age of 45 will need a different mix and volume of services than will a population that has an average age of 65.

The principal advantage an HMO offers is that it can offer very tight cost controls while providing broad-based health care services to subscribers. HMOs operate in an extremely rigid business fashion. These tight controls, however, have been criticized by some as leading to inflexible utilization policies. Because they take the risk for paying for health care services, HMOs also take the opportunity to get close to making or encouraging medical decisions for their physicians. Their policies govern which physicians patients may see, what tests and procedures can be certified, what facilities patients may use, and when patients may seek advice or treatment from specialists. These are decisions that used to be the unquestioned domain of physicians; the fact that, in part, managers are making them is causing much serious public concern.

HMOs control costs for services provided by keeping tight reins on:

- Inpatient hospital services
- Outpatient services
- Doctor visits
- Use of specialists
- Diagnostic testing

By enrolling a large number of subscribers, HMOs can take advantage of economies of scale, which benefits the HMO by lowering its average cost per subscriber. HMOs are also able to operate with reduced administrative costs.

As one might expect, one of the principal criticisms of HMOs is their use of such tight controls and their limiting of patient access to services and physicians. Some people are concerned that they cannot see their traditional family doctors because their HMOs do not have their physicians under contract. Despite these criticisms and other complaints, the growth of HMOs has been rapid. HMO enrollment in 1970 was 3 million. In 1980 enrollment increased to 9 million; 38 million in 1992, and 42 million in 1994, when approximately 16% of the population was enrolled in HMO plans (Fig. 5-3A,B).

Administrative Efforts by HMOs to Control Their Costs

Other cost-saving measures are accomplished by HMO nursing personnel auditing and documenting the utilization elements noted below:

- Admission and discharge dates
- Timeliness of tests versus date of results
- Effectiveness of treatment
- Who ordered diagnostic tests and how
- Number of repeated tests or procedures
- Type and frequency of complications
- Appropriateness of tests
- Effectiveness and timeliness of discharge planning
- Paying *only* for services provided

HMOs put great emphasis on the fact that the primary care physician (PCP) manages each patient's episode of care. It is generally held that approximately 80% of hosptial costs, for example, are generated by the physician's pen when ordering tests and treatment regimens. This physician is responsible directly to the HMO for monitoring and documenting the patient's progress, tests, diagnosis, and treatment throughout each episode of care. The primary care physician is also responsible for coordinating patient referrals to specialists. Controlling costs associated with use of specialists is a very important part of HMO cost control programs. Fees charged by specialists can be 50% to 100% higher than those

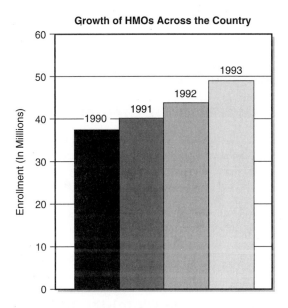

▶ FIGURE 5-3 Illustrates HMO penetration as of 1993 and growth over recent years.

charged by primary care physicians. This simple formula is a method for benchmarking an appropriate number of referrals to specialist physicians:

$$\frac{\text{Number of referrals}}{\text{Per 100 cases seen by PCP}} = \text{Referral rate}$$

For example:

$$\frac{11 \text{ referrals}}{100 \text{ patients}} = 11 \% \text{ referral rate}$$

Most HMOs require that a patient has an authorization form before he or she can see a specialist, regardless of the patient's wishes. In other words, some HMOs will not pay the fee if one of its patients independently sees a specialist. Further, if the specialist orders tests or procedures without the PCP's authorization the HMO will usually not pay. On the other hand, HMOs may require a second opinion when one of their patients faces a significant treatment plan or surgery. They view the second opinion as a money saving measure providing protection against unnecessary, costly treatments. Another important cost-saving philosophy held by HMOs is the belief that effective education and preventive health care programs yield significant long-term benefits to both the patient and the HMO's bottom line.

HMOs may be either open- or closed-panel organizations. Open-panel HMOs may contract with private physicians, while closed-panel HMOs only employ their own physicians and refer patients out only after following strict guidelines. The significance of this difference to the patient is two-fold. First, the degree of personal choice a patient might have to see or not to see a physician is affected. Second, it is commonly understood that physicians who are fully employed by an HMO may not have as much freedom of choice in prescribing treatment, medication, or testing as a private physician has. The closed-panel format sometimes places more restrictions on both the patient and the physician as they make judgments.

HMOs are regulated like any other insurance company by their states' insurance commissioners and are subject to prevailing restrictions and requirements. The influence of HMOs has increased significantly throughout the country (Fig. 5-3).

IMPACT THAT HMOs HAVE HAD ON HEALTH CARE COSTS

HMOs must show sensitivity to the quality of services that they offer patients. Quality is in many instances evaluated on the basis of the patient's perception and includes factors such as access, timeliness, accuracy, appropriateness, and the manner with which services are provided. In addition, the patient's overall perception of final outcome weighs significantly.

HMOs have their own boards of directors and well-defined boards of medical directors and management staffs. The exact structure may vary from one HMO to another. Their business strategies also vary somewhat depending on their tax statuses. They follow basic peer review procedures for all physicians they have, whether the physician is fully employed and salaried or under a provider contract.

PHOs: PHYSICIAN-HOSPITAL ORGANIZATIONS

Another managed care format involves the establishment of a nonprofit corporation by the medical staff of a single hospital or of a group of hospitals; these hospitals then function in effect as a limited HMO. This organization is referred to as a PHO (physician-hospital organization). The PHO can contract with employers in the community just as any other HMO might do. This nonprofit corporation is very similar in nature to a nonprofit HMO and must conform to all standard rules of incorporation. The board of directors is composed of key hospital administrators and representatives of the medical staff. The PHO will enter into agreements in which it promises to provide full coverage to employers' subscribers. If it cannot provide certain services, the PHO will refer patients to another facility at no additional cost to the patient or employer.

PPOs: PREFERRED PROVIDER ORGANIZATIONS

Preferred provider organizations are variations on HMOs. PPOs are groups of providers (not necessarily hospital-based) who group together as a corporation to enter into contractual agreements with individuals or groups to provide health care services. Such providers often include groups of physicians and facilities that, compared to many HMOs, offer the patient much more choice of physicians and facilities.

WHO IS COVERED?

A survey done in 1990 found that approximately 42% of the country's corporations offered group health insurance coverage to their employees. This means that the remaining population is either not insured, underinsured, or is covered by individual plans for which people pay themselves. The Medicare law requires open enrollment periods during the year. During these periods, any person who meets the criteria to receive Medicare benefits may apply and be granted coverage. Figure 5-4 shows a broader distribution of funds.

CAPITATION OF HEALTH CARE SERVICES

Capitation is viewed differently by payers and providers. From the payer's perspective, future expenses can be estimated from actuarial tables that are becoming more and more accurate. From the provider's perspective, risk is increased. In fact, under a capitated payment system, the fewer patients there are to diagnose, and treat, the more profit the provider takes in because it still receives the amount the contract specifies. All services are covered by that annual amount. In fact, the provider's best operating scenario is that it sees no patients at all for the entire period of the contract. In most instances the provider receives regular payments on the basis of $ per member/month as we saw earlier in Table 5-1.

A health care system with open access that utilizes advanced technology and protocols is inherently very expensive. This is especially true when the patient's primary consultant (the physician) and provider (hospital or office) are paid on a fee for service basis by a third party. In addition, it has been shown that increased availability, achieved either by reducing patient out-of-pocket expenses and/or by increasing services' convenience, generates increased demand; this elevates cost even further. Using multiple research studies, health care economists have shown payment models that provide revenue to providers without imposing tough monitoring definitely encourage and increase demand for additional services. Yet, limiting funds for services provided by facilities is potentially dangerous.

Health care reform of the future, whether it is caused by private industry efforts or by government legislation, will be successful only if prudent criteria for payment are established. We have seen that health care administrators of the past were probably not business-minded enough; we must now be careful to guard against the possibility that the business-people who are today determining much about how medicine is practiced will cause even more pain by starving the health care system of cash.

RECENT LEGISLATION AND GOVERNMENT MONITORING OF HEALTH CARE

The first major legislation in recent times was designed to effectively control health care expenses came into effect when President Reagan signed the prospective payment system into law in 1983. This landmark legislation forever changed Medicare system reimbursement to health care providers and provided a clear sign of the future for non-Medicare reimbursement as well. The groups who pay most U.S. health care costs are:

1. The federal government
2. State governments through Medicare and Medicaid
3. Employers through benefit packages to employees
4. Out-of-pocket payment from patients

In many instances, reduced cost offer less variety of services, and in some instances, they limit access by not paying for certain procedures. In some cases, people who fit certain profiles, such as nonsmokers, are charged lower premiums. People with disorders, diseases, or other health conditions might have to pay very high insurance premiums or will experience rationing. Our culture has not to date accepted rationing as a reasonable alternative; however, continued cost-cutting efforts and capitated rates could push us dangerously close to rationing. Also, there is a very subtle threshold that separates tight economic controls from rationing, and perhaps the general public would have trouble distinguishing one from the

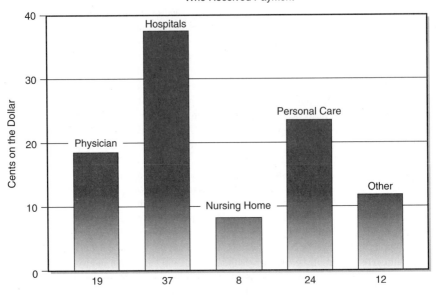

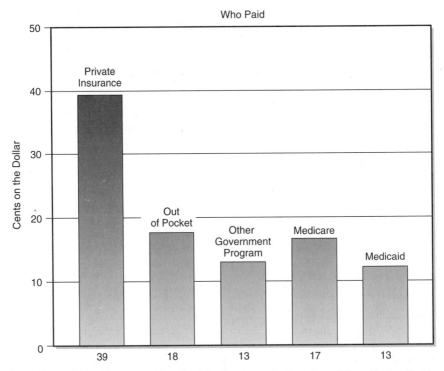

▶ **FIGURE 5−4** Shows distribution of recipients and sources of health care dollars. (Source: Health Care Financing Administration, Office of the Actuary.)

other. How can a health program providing high-quality services and acceptable access be developed at the national level and not lead to excessive costs or rationing? Washington has been working on this question without answering it since the early 1900s, and in this vacuum, the private managed health care organizations emerged. Four possible answers to this question have been considered:

- Increase government subsidies from funds that are perceived to be less critical to the country's well-being.
- Create a strongly competitive environment that includes the carriers, physicians, and providers.
- Increase government regulation to root out waste in the system.
- Develop a system having very little government intervention, and simply let the market find its own level of supply and demand for services at nonregulated prices.

It is clear that none of these answers alone could have solved the entire problem. Although both payers and providers can see the popularity and benefits of managed care organizations, questions regarding the long-term effect of this revolution will have to be answered. It is very easy for the payer to say services are covered or provided. The *degree* or level to which these services are covered is a very different matter that can have an unexpected and surprising effect on the patient's actual level of access to the service.

The first step toward answering the access–quality question is having a clear definition for access to service that U.S. citizens will accept. There is still little agreement on this definition. In fact, as U.S. legislators work on a new national health plan, I believe that most U.S. citizens are only vaguely aware of what might actually be at stake with regards to their future access and limitations of coverage. A national plan that is designed to include approximately 40 million more people at no or very little additional cost to the government seems unrealistic unless access for the average individual who is currently insured is reduced.

One element that has been consistent in all successful insurance plans, whether private or government-based, is that a broad base of insurance subscribers is necessary to pay enough premiums into the system to support the relatively few people who will need health care. Therefore, any successful national health plan will have to have a very large number of subscribers with a very wide range of age groups.

It will also become more and more important for individuals to plan and implement savings programs early in life so that they will have sufficient funds to supplement whatever health care plan is in effect when they reach a mature age. This may require a thorough reconsideration of personal spending philosophies and a reallocation of personal funds because even the most humanistic national plan may not cover all health services that will be desired in the future.

From the physician's point of view, national health plans may have other disadvantages. In these plans, physicians fear a loss of reasonable flexibility to exercise alternatives for tests and treatment. Some believe that the lack of fee-for-service incentives to physicians will seriously affect their professionalism and effort, and many physicians say that this may be true to some degree. Such changes are certainly not to be taken lightly, but, over time, a new generation of physicians will come into medicine and learn to be productive and effective under a salary system. Whether physicians' performance will suffer will in part be determined by our culture's expectations. The greater danger may lie in placing too stringent limitations on physicians' ability to prescribe tests and treatment plans for their patients.

OVERMANAGING COSTS

There is an old adage that too much of a good thing is not good. In the context of managed care, there is the danger that if payments to providers on a per-member per-month basis are too low, a line will eventually be crossed such that short-term savings will occur but so will increased long-term costs. We should be mindful that hidden costs may lurk in subtly decreasing services to patients. HMOs will be under increasing scrutiny as they establish criteria that justify not paying for services to their subscribers. This may be especially true among the for-profit HMOs, which are in the business to make profits for their shareholders.

Contracts that are negotiated by payers include criteria that define authorized and nonauthorized services. If a test, medication, treatment, or other service is provided to a patient that does not fit those criteria, the HMO will refuse to pay for it. Setting such criteria is certainly a double-edged sword—it can reduce unnecessary services and expenses; however, it can also set inappropriate limitations on access to health care if the criteria are enforced too rigidly. Thus, the cost of patient care may be temporarily postponed or hidden.

The notion of dealing with hidden costs comes into play when appropriate physician options are removed or severely limited, and recurrences, complications, and the like subsequently result which can be much more costly both in dollars and in a patient's well-being. History shows that when one looks at HMOs' data regarding recurrent problems, readmissions, complications, and the like, they are not significantly different from those of more traditional payers. We must be careful as a nation not to loose sight of certain benchmarks that will help us to keep our current standards of care.

S T U D Y   Q U E S T I O N S

1. Briefly explain basic differences between the payers below:

   Commercial insurance companies
   Blue Cross
   HMOs
   The federal government

2. Provide a brief summary of how health care services were paid for during the following periods: mid-1700s to 1800; 1800 to 1900; 1900 to the present.

3. In what year and area of health care did the United States government first significantly influence payment toward the cost of medical services?

4. Give three examples of how the Social Security Act of 1964 affected health care costs and availability of services. Which group of people benefitted the most from this legislation?

5. Review the rate of inflation of health care costs against the rate of growth of the GNP over the last 10 years. Why do you think it is important to keep an acceptable ratio between the GNP and health care costs?

6. What are the positive and negative aspects of managed care? What segments of our population do you think favor managed care and which do not, and why?

7. What is cost loading and how did this affect charges for hospital services? Were there alternative methods that could have been considered?

8. Write a one-page summary that expresses the dilemma involved in providing

high availability and quality of health care service to the general population at an affordable cost.

9. Write a brief summary that expresses the advantages and cautions that should be considered when developing alternatives or substitutions for providing health care services so that costs can be reduced.

10. As an administrator, what strategies would you expect your chief financial officer to recommend to maximize the financial bottom line with respect to payer mix, patient days, length of stay, quality of service, availability of service to everyone in the community, and maintaining employee morale?

11. Describe the effect our third-party payer system has on overall health care costs and what you would propose as an alternative.

12. As the CEO of your hospital, what strategy would you want to use when negotiating with a health maintenance organization considering a large contract with your institution?

Quality of Care

OBJECTIVES FOR STUDY

After reading this chapter, the student will

▶ Appreciate the scope of effort required to develop and maintain a hospital-wide quality assurance program.

▶ Understand the need for continuous quality improvement programs to meet patient care needs and regulatory requirements.

▶ Appreciate the role of a hospital's quality assurance department and how the requirements of the Joint Commission on Accreditation of Health Organizations have changed over recent years.

▶ Appreciate the role of the radiology department's CQI program for improving services and the need to integrate its program with the central hospital program.

▶ Understand the role of peer review programs and how they affect patient care and outcome of services.

▶ Understand how the prospective payment system affects quality of patient care and the scope of services offered to patients.

THE QUALITY MANAGEMENT DEPARTMENT

The greatest impact that the changing payer environment has had in recent years on the health care industry falls into two distinct areas of quality; quality of care and appropriateness of services provided, and outcome assessment. Quality of care is practiced and is the responsibility of individuals who are encouraged and supported by the hospital through proper direction and adequate resources. Many hospitals today utilize their Quality Management Departments and subsidiaries (individual departments of the hospital) to carry the overall responsibility for coordinating and driving this effort. This is certainly one of the most challenging responsibilities in health care today. The difficulty of the job lies in the need to coordinate enormous amounts of detailed information and activities among ALL departments on an ongoing basis. The scope of elements that need to be analyzed and tracked through multiple stages of development and implementation within a hospital make this a daunting undertaking. Some of these elements are:

- Appropriateness of service provided
- Outcome: how successful were the results of services provided?
- Efficacy: the cost-effectiveness of services or equipment relative to the medical outcome the patient expected
- Documentation
- Process: assessment and improvement
- Safety: equipment, personnel, patients, facilities, supplies
- Timeliness of service: scheduling delays, report turnaround, total time needed to produce the expected medical result

Making this mission even more complicated, the scope of responsibility also includes monitoring the activities of private physicians who are the engines for bringing patients into the system for care. Physicians tend to place a high value on functioning as individuals and are less comfortable when working in a structured environment. They are in fact trained in part to be self-reliant and are expected to make decisions as quickly as possible. This, combined with their political strength as the hospital's primary source of patient referrals, adds leverage to their demands for independence. This model, however, is changing as health care moves toward managed care.

We will focus on the hospital's Quality Management Department in this chapter by describing some of its primary functions. We will also discuss worthwhile characteristics of a radiology department's continuous quality improvement (CQI) program. As we go along, we should keep in mind that each department must have its own quality management program with defined efforts toward continuous quality improvement (CQI).

The mission of the Quality Management Department at the institutional level is to monitor the appropriateness, effectiveness, and quality of patient care. This may seem to be a relatively straightforward undertaking because everyone claims this universal goal. However, it requires developing an effective and comprehensive list of reports and statistics which provide indications about the effectiveness of care from the perspectives of equipment, facility, personnel utilization, cost, and the quality of management within the institution. The hospital's quality assurance department fundamentally acts as a clearing house for activities that impact quality, appropriateness, and effectiveness of care. It also takes on the role of facilitator in many instances to develop and advocate initiatives for overall hospital and department processes.

In the past, the typical approach to quality of care was different than it has become over the last few years. The criteria used by the JCAHO until the mid-1980s were task-oriented and they outlined fairly specific objectives that were written along department lines. These criteria resulted in heightened awareness of quality of care because they focused mainly on establishing and documenting procedures. They did not emphasize effectiveness or outcome of care to the extent that we see today. Nor did they emphasize the need for improvement plans that include the participation of multidisciplinary groups to solve quality of service issues across department lines. In almost all cases, the use of a multidisciplinary group is vital to the analysis of a given operational issue in any given department.

MOVING FROM YESTERDAY'S TO TODAY'S QUALITY MANAGEMENT

In the past, primary attention was aimed at the mechanics of defining, preparing, and following procedures that were expected to impact patient care. Huge amounts of time were spent on documentation, and less emphasis was placed on how a service specifically benefitted the patient. These efforts were also quarantined into departmental boxes. The philosophy was that if department procedures were established and followed, patient care would improve. As a result, the period from the late 1970s to the mid-1980s saw more and better policies and procedures being written. Feedback mechanisms from each department to the hospital's "QA" department were also implemented, and everyone began talking about improving the quality of care through these policies. Unfortunately, this effort was directed toward developing policies and tracking how well these policies and procedures were being observed.

Today, the emphasis on documenting policies and procedures has given way to an emphasis on outcome assessment. This approach focuses primary energy on patient management, with an emphasis on assessing actual results of the services that have been provided. Methods for measuring complications, continuity of care, timeliness, and the appropriateness of services are today themselves measured against new outcome criteria. This change in focus is significant, because these outcome criteria are not only established by individual departments, they are also reviewed and in many instances managed by multidisciplinary focus groups or task groups that directly involve several different departments. This change in focus is also significant because problem solving becomes a hospital-wide effort: procedures are forced to change across department lines rather than in just one department working alone to meet the outcome required by the organization. In addition the role and individual responsibility of each employee takes on more significance within the hospital's overall Quality of Care Program. Problem analysis and resolution accomplished through a multidisciplinary panel provides a more comprehensive approach. Figure 6-1 shows the traditional department improvement process, which forces change to occur vertically rather than horizontally.

QUALITY MANAGEMENT

Quality management was also introduced with greater emphasis. It addresses the actual complexity of problems from the perspective of how well management function. We will emphasize in Chapter Nine that the quality and style of a hospital's management has a huge impact on quality of care and services provided. Therefore, a CQI program must include improvements along a broad range of management techniques.

The new philosophies of outcome assessment, multidisciplinary task groups, and quali-

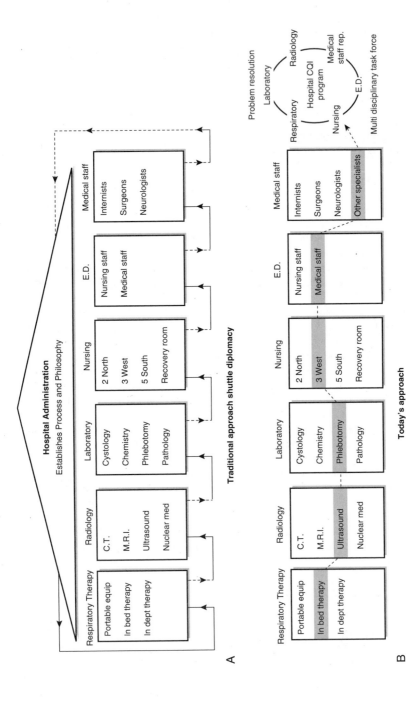

▶ **FIGURE 6–1** (A) Illustrates the traditional approach to solving operational problems. (B) Demonstrates the structure of a CQI multidisciplinary problem-solving task force. The approach today emphasizes getting the people who actually do the work to participate directly in the process of evaluating current problems and designing new, improved processes. This change often utilizes the department director as a contact person who mainly functions as an adviser and as someone who can enforce the proposed changes rather than as the designer of the plan.

ty management caused important movements toward team analysis and program implementation and away from each department individually defining criteria, analyzing present conditions, and implementing changes for improvement. In today's model, the complexities of providing care are given more appropriate recognition, and the basic challenge with this in mind is to find ways to improve outcome of the services provided.

In Figure 6-1, we see a model that helps describe today's approach. This generally leads to more appropriate and effective solutions or outcomes of service. Frustration lies, however, in the fact that analyzing and developing new procedures by using multidisciplinary groups often takes considerably longer than the old approach. This is particularly true when people believe that they already know the answer and exactly how to proceed with implementing the solution.

GROUP-ORIENTED PROBLEM SOLVING

In a growing number of hospitals, multidisciplinary panels are likely to include representatives from nursing, respiratory medicine, food services, central transportation, and pathology in order to develop effective patient-focused outcome criteria. This team will also evaluate and track specific elements of care over time. In almost every situation, only when such a team of people meets to discuss a problem does the full complexity of the circumstances surface.

Let's look at an example. The radiology department is having difficulty getting patients on time from a particular nursing floor. The initial assumption was that the nursing floor was not well organized or didn't really want to extend sufficient effort to help solve what used to be considered radiology's problem. The approach now is that radiology's problem also becomes the patient's problem. Multidisciplinary groups are needed to find solutions to the higher level of integration of services and the dependencies that lead to effective outcomes. The dependencies have always been there; however, we are now learning how to integrate efforts from several dependent departments to arrive at the best solution possible. Anything less will result in overall institutional inefficiencies that we can no longer afford. In this case, the problem actually involved several elements which were not all governed by the nurse manager. In addition, it was necessary to have the dietary, respiratory, and physical medicine departments participate in a more thorough review of the circumstances that contributed to the delays. Without this multidisciplinary approach and some open discussion on the matter, the problem would have been only partially solved, and continued frustration between radiology and the nursing floor would have occurred.

▶ TABLE 6-1

REDUCED DELAYS PRODUCED BY MULTIDISCIPLINARY PROCESS IMPROVEMENT TEAM TIME INTERVALS BELOW IN MINUTES

	OVERALL TIME PT WAS IN ED	PT ENTERED ED TO PT LEAVING X-RAY EXPOSURE RM	TIME X-RAY PLACED TO TIME PT ENTERED EXPOSURE RM
Initial results	111	98	20
Six months follow-up	87	78	9
Net improvement	21.6%	20.4%	55.0%

Shows results of a multidisciplinary team effort to reduce waiting periods for emergency patients. After several meetings held to evaluate data from a wide range of operations criteria, a better understanding of critical path activities by the ED and Radiology helped pave the way for overall system improvements.

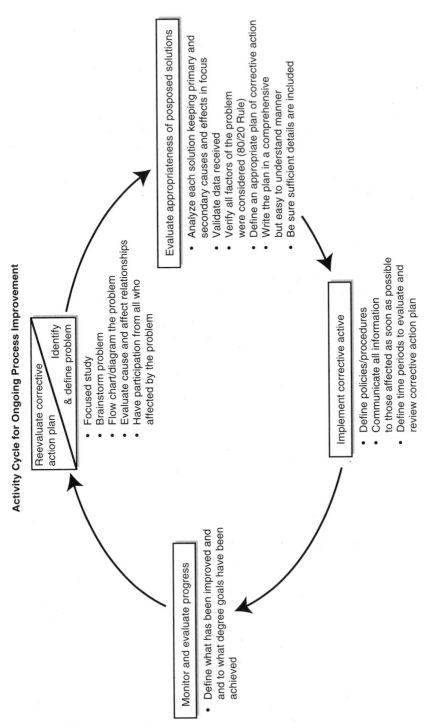

Activity Cycle for Ongoing Process Improvement

Reevaluate corrective action plan

Identify & define problem
- Focused study
- Brainstorm problem
- Flow chart/diagram the problem
- Evaluate cause and affect relationships
- Have participation from all who affected by the problem

Evaluate appropriateness of posposed solutions
- Analyze each solution keeping primary and secondary causes and effects in focus
- Validate data received
- Verify all factors of the problem were considered (80/20 Rule)
- Define an appropriate plan of corrective action
- Write the plan in a comprehensive but easy to understand manner
- Be sure sufficient details are included

Implement corrective active
- Define policies/procedures
- Communicate all information to those affected as soon as possible
- Define time periods to evaluate and review corrective action plan

Monitor and evaluate progress
- Define what has been improved and and to what degree goals have been achieved

▶ **FIGURE 6-2** Shows the concept of the CQI process and philosophy, which require continually evaluating solutions, measuring their effectiveness, and re-designing processes/operations.

A second example of this type of approach occurred when Radiology could not provide fast enough turnaround time for stat portable studies. A work group that included nursing, radiology, a representative physician, and the quality management department developed a much more structured process that improved the situation substantially. The process included a clear airing of all perceived problems from the participants. This led to a mandate by all to do a detailed and comprehensive survey, which provided very meaningful data. The result was a buy-in from everyone involved, and the procedure for ordering and providing the service changed substantially. In addition, a much more meaningful understanding of each department's legitimate expectations can be developed (Fig. 6-4).

A final example involves a thorough investigation of turnaround time for radiology studies ordered by the Emergency Department (ED). The process included an open discussion of perceived issues, which was followed by a plan for improvement. Table 6-1 shows the progress that was made as a result. In addition, other issues were discussed and resolved that improved operations in both departments.

Experience has shown that all new programs, procedures, and protocols must be monitored closely after the implementation phase. Often the level of attention and effort needed to support and maintain the effectiveness of newly implemented continuous quality improvement (CQI) and critical path processes and procedures is significantly underestimated. If they are not monitored closely by a *designated* person or persons their long term effectiveness and efficiencies will surely diminish. Cooperating departments with the best intentions often lose sight of subtle slippage. One of the fundamental problems is that these subtle slippages are often viewed as acceptable postimplementation adjustments that may be necessary. However, if they go unnoticed, they broaden over time and can evolve into a more generalized system problem that becomes at least as problematic as the concerns that were initially addressed. Periodic meeting times are needed with both managers and line employees to assess and critique what has been happening and, if necessary, to consider adjustments as needed.

CONTINUOUS QUALITY IMPROVEMENT (CQI)

The effort does not stop, however, at maintaining acceptable performance standards; there is an emphasis on continuous improvement. The process of continuous quality improvement should involve at minimum the functions listed below:

1. Formation of group/committee to review key department criteria
2. Evaluate performance against these criteria
3. Determine opportunities to increase criteria or standards
4. Develop and implement plans for improvement
5. Monitor results
6. Make adjustments as needed to meet revised criteria

A diagram of the continuous quality improvement process is shown in Figure 6-2. In theory, activities identified around this circle are continually repeated until there is no reasonable opportunity for further improvement. We may also discontinue further efforts when it appears that further effort will yield fewer results than if another problem is addressed. When an acceptable level of effectiveness or outcome of service is reached for an appropriate period of time, the work team may declare mission accomplished. It is then the responsibility of the department to identify other elements to be improved. CQI programs require a high degree of commitment and a comprehensive effort, but the benefits can have a significant effect on all departments within a hospital. Figure 6-3 outlines the chain

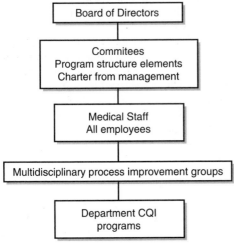

Strong Commitment and Direction from Senior Management

Board of Directors

Commitees
Program structure elements
Charter from management

Medical Staff
All employees

Multidisciplinary process improvement groups

Department CQI
programs

▶ **FIGURE 6–3** Structure of a hospital's CQI program. These programs show considerable variety in structure among hospitals. The key elements include a sincere commitment by senior managers to encourage interdisciplinary focus groups to work effectively.

of responsibility that is necessary to maintain an effective CQI program throughout the hospital.

THE JOINT COMMISSION ON ACCREDITATION OF HEALTH CARE ORGANIZATIONS (JCAHO)

As part of the Medicare legislation of 1964, the federal government, through the Health Care Finance Administration (HCFA), created an agent to directly monitor and evaluate the quality and cost-effectiveness of medical services delivered by facilities that receive Medicare patients. This agent is known as the Joint Commission on Accreditation of Health Care Organizations (JCAHO) and has the charge to develop methods and parameters used to assess the quality of care provided in the hospitals and to credential those hospitals that meet these criteria. It also has the charge to define a process that assures ongoing evaluation of quality improvement of hospital services. The JCAHO has had significant clout due to its authority to withhold credentials from hospitals because of noncompliance with its criteria. If a hospital does not receive accreditation by this organization, its Medicare reimbursementis threatened. Losing this percentage of overall revenue would be catastrophic for any hospital's financial status.

THE JCAHO SURVEY FORMAT

Hospitals are surveyed by the JCAHO through in-depth audits of hospital records. These surveys are conducted by multidisciplinary teams of health care professionals usually consisting of a nurse, a physician, and a hospital administrator.

The survey team will typically visit a hospital for approximately three days. In that time, each member of the survey team reviews designated areas of the hospital. The nurse, for example, will be primarily interested in the nursing department, medical records, and the facility's utilization review procedures. The physician will spend much of his or her time

Analysis of Stat Portable Delays

	Time ordered to time scheduled	Time scheduled to time technician received order	Time technician relieved order until entered in computer	Time entered in computer computer gen request	Time technician required to reach portable equipment	Continued as needed....
Minutes	10	5	4	2	25	→

Portable Turnaround Analysis
Identification of Time Gates

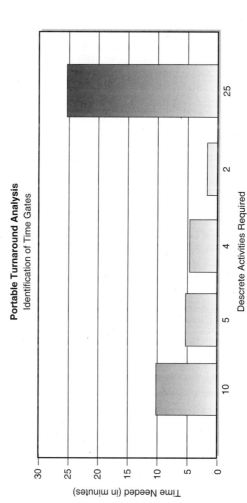

▶ **FIGURE 6-4** Illustrates that, of the five specific activities shown, only one has a dramatic effect on the problem. Therefore, the effort needed to solve the problem must be applied accordingly. This illustration describes a relatively simple problem. As the complexity of operational issues increases and the need for establishing critical paths also increases, it becomes more difficult to identify and evaluate how each discrete activity contributes to the problem. The 80/20 rule has great application in these circumstances.

reviewing medical staff credentialling records, physician credentialling procedures, and the various clinical departments and may also participate in medical records assessment. The administrator will evaluate administrative and support services such as equipment safety policies, maintenance, and environmental services. Hospitals are generally surveyed every three years. Some hospitals require annual reviews because of unsatisfactory findings.

The survey is generally scheduled several months in advance, although unannounced surveys are possible. A scheduled survey may be preceded by several months of notifications regarding new and revised guidelines, recommendations, and expectations that are described in detailed and expansive booklets. In effect, each department must provide assurances to the survey team that it is functioning in concert with these guidelines and has been providing appropriate documentation of effective outcome-oriented patient care initiatives. Another group of elements that the JCAHO has especially emphasized, is the matter of equipment safety and maintenance.

OVERVIEW OF THE JCAHO PROGRAM

The JCAHO produces a manual which contains comprehensive and detailed instructions and recommendations that are the basis for evaluating the level of patient care that is provided in a hospital. This manual has changed dramatically over the last several years in terms of both content and scope. Currently, the JCAHO has divided the care provided in a hospital into four sections:

▶ **Section 1: Care of the patient**
   Assessment of the patient
   Treatment of the patient, tests, meds, diag., etc.
   Operative and other invasive procedures
   Education of patient and family
   Rights of patients and organizational efforts
   Entry to settings or service
   Nutritional care
   Coordination of care

▶ **Section 2: Organizational function**
   Leadership
   Management of information
   Improving organizational performance

▶ **Section 3: Structures with important functions**
   Governing body
   Management and administration
   Medical staff
   Nursing

▶ **Section 4: Other department/service specific requirements**
   Hospital sponsored ambulatory care service
   Medical records service
   Medical staff
   Patient and family education
   Professional library and health information

Quality assessment and improvement
Responsibilities of department service directors
Surgical/anesthesia services
Utilization review

As you can see, these sections deal with specific issues within an aspect of patient care provided by the hospital. Each of these sections affects all departments within the hospital, and each department must therefore address contribution or role in each of these categories. This approach gives great encouragement to the development of multidisciplinary groups to solve problems.

The JCAHO has also defined a framework for improving organizational performance to help establish an overall environment within the organization that will support the effort of continued quality improvement. This is another incentive to use a multidisciplinary approach to patient-focused care. To encourage use of this framework, the JCAHO has advocated *internal attributes* which they say must be present and evident for a hospital to achieve high overall performance standards. These internal attributes are the basis for the current emphasis on quality management:

- Leadership
- Management of human resources
- Management of information
- Improving organizational performance

When put into practice, these attributes define a framework for more uniform, system-oriented improvement efforts. Such application requires a level of research, investigation, documentation, and monitoring that is characteristic of scientific methodology, which should be supported by quality management efforts throughout the hospital. There is no specific point at which these efforts begin or end, but rather a continual effort by various departments working together to achieve a given element of outcome for diagnosis or treatment services.

JCAHO STANDARDS

To provide further assurance that problems are reviewed and corrected in a programmatic fashion, the JCAHO has advocated the continuous improvement cycle approach, presented in Figure 6-2. CQI teams will use several different techniques for researching and analyzing problems, including:

- Open discussion of possible solutions (brainstorming)
- Flow charting
- Defining discrete cause and effect scenarios
- Researching statistics from outside sources
- Commissioning direct patient inquiries

The importance of performing these detailed investigative and analytical efforts cannot be underestimated. To illustrate this, you should review a flowchart that was used to define decision points and impasses to help identify solutions for providing stat portable X-ray exams. As you review Figure 6-1, consider the number of discussions that might be important to have with nursing personnel, aides, physicians, and technologists before all related information can be placed on the table. Then consider the probability of one person understanding the implications of all related activities.

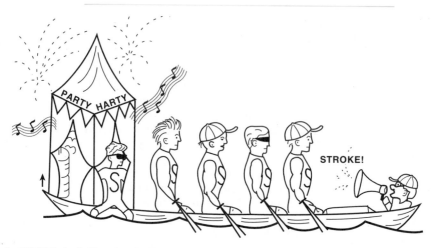

▶ **FIGURE 6-5** Illustrates the 80/20 rule. Note that 20% of the factors have caused 80% or more of the problem.

On the other hand, a balance between reality and the pursuit of perfection must be maintained to accomplish anything meaningful. Therefore, the 80/20 rule should be considered. The 80/20 principle or rule was first described at the turn of the century by the economist Vilfredo Pareto (Fig. 6-6). The principle was later applied to management issues by Juran, who cautioned against investing a significant amount of resources to address less important matters. Loosely stated, the principle says that about 20% of factors contribute to 80% of a problem. Therefore, in many instances, it is more worthwhile to identify that 20% than to investigate and try to fix all the factors leading to a problem. Keeping the 80/20 rule in mind, one may use a bar graph, as shown in Figure 6-4 to demonstrate the relative impact each element has on the whole problem.

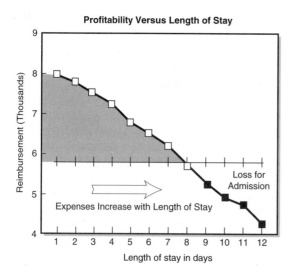

▶ **FIGURE 6-6** Demonstrates the concept of profitability relative to length of stay with prospective capitated reimbursement.

THE PROCESS OF PEER REVIEW

PROs have developed more and more sophisticated methods for monitoring the efficiency and efficacy of hospital services ordered by physicians. This monitoring occurs through a process of audits which are conducted at the hospital by representatives from the PRO office by the hospital's medical staff and administration. During this audit, any number of patient charts may be reviewed at random and to any degree of detail the reviewers feel is appropriate. In many hospitals, the process is monitored through the hospital's quality management department. Physicians who use more resources than the norm to reach a diagnosis are being identified in virtually every hospital today. As a result, all hospitals have developed internal medical audit and utilization review departments.

The mandate from the federal government to monitor appropriateness and cost-effectiveness of care provided is delegated to the states, which administer the PRO audits. If these audits indicate that appropriate care was not provided, the auditors have the authority to disallow a portion or all of the Medicare or Medicaid payments associated with that admission. The AMA points out five basic elements that are important for PRO programs:

1. Direct and concurrent observation of physician performance. This emphasis is on the capacity of the physician to blend good analytical ability with professional knowledge.

2. A screening system that measures all care given against known outcome. This system consists of internal audits accomplished by nurses and MDs who agree to serve in such a capacity. Physicians often express objections to this system on the basis it amounts to "big brothering."

3. An appropriate method of rationing the auditing effort to fit circumstances that are worthy of review (rather than mass reviews of a large number of medical records) should be in place.

4. Sufficient and intelligent exception allowances must be built into the criteria to account for situations that do not fall into the norm.

5. The audit must include a method for aggregating the various decisions or points of care documented in a medical record so that they can be compared easily with established trends. This information should also be worked into an information pool to help future decisions.

DEVELOPING A PEER REVIEW PLAN

The development of a peer review plan cannot occur rapidly. The AMA describes four stages that the process usually passes through. These include the development of a positive view of the program by physicians. Links between levels of training, skill, expense, and ordering criteria are described and defined. Provisional monitoring criteria for new staff members involve practice standards, which include such elements as the number and complexity of cases handled by a physician and timeliness of diagnosis and treatment. Other phases of development establish consultation efforts that encourage a format for working with auditors to analyze physicians' performance and finally, for investigative monitoring, which involves retrospectively researching current indicators of questionable care.

Participating in these initiatives takes a substantial amount of physicians' time: Time given to routine meetings and to serving on program design and development committees has substantially increased. In addition, stress levels increase when there are frequent meetings regarding protocols that control virtually every medical decision made by the physician. In fact, in most hospitals, each physician's performance is now measured against indicators in the categories below:

- Length of stay
- Overall cost of case generated
- Breakout of cost for treatment, medication, and tests
- Number of cases that failed a review
- Corrective action taken after physician notification
- Suspension because of poor review
- Timeliness of diagnosis
- Surgical time
- Accuracy rate of diagnosis
- Rate of complications
- Mortality rate

THE APPEAL PROCESS

Even with the best peer review programs, there is the potential for errors in judging physician performance. Performance profiles can be deceptive, and an appropriate review process must be in place to give physicians the opportunity to clarify erroneous reports. Sometimes physician evaluations and even practice credentials may be impacted by these reports. In this event, an appeal process is required. Such an appeal process would include:

- A fair hearing
- A timely hearing
- A judicial process
- Attorney representation

EVALUATION OF THE REVIEWERS/AUDITORS

It is equally important to monitor and evaluate the auditors who produce utilization and physician performance reports. The elements below show some criteria for evaluating reviewers:

- Delayed reviews
- Superficial reviews
- Under/overevaluation
- Projected responsibility
- Reviewer incompetence to review medical records

To guard against the above problems, reviewers must be adequately trained and then monitored to detect any misses and inappropriate "calls" that they make. The operational costs associated with developing hospital-based medical audit programs has risen substantially over recent years.

DOCUMENTATION, DOCUMENTATION, DOCUMENTATION, AND STATISTICS

Documentation has clearly been one of the keys to meeting standards imposed by regulators on the one hand and payers on the other. Often, reimbursement denials are actually the result of poor documentation rather than of improperly provided or inappropriate service. Administrators therefore have good reason to apply strong pressure on physicians to comply with all regulations, patient management protocols, and documentation procedures.

WHO AUTHORIZES PATIENT ADMISSION?

One of the most striking examples of the need for documentation is the preadmission process. Previously, a physician with admission privileges would be able to admit a patient when he or she felt it was medically indicated. Preadmission protocol would have the physician simply write orders for tests needed and call the admitting office for a bed. Under today's more restrictive reimbursement, utilization, and peer review criteria, physicians may not admit their patients until a thorough and predefined preadmission work-up has been completed. In most instances, payers have developed individual preadmission "certification" criteria that must be followed to the letter by the hospital's preadmission review process. Considering that a community hospital may have 15,000 admissions per year, even a small percentage of denied payments could impact its annual fiscal status. (See Figs. 2-6 and 2-7.) The risk of loosing even a small percentage of these admissions because of poor documentation or not following admission criteria could noticeably impact the hospital's bottom line.

EVALUATING PATIENT CARE UNDER THE PROSPECTIVE PAYMENT SYSTEM

When patients are admitted, their medical work-ups lead to designating a Diagnostic Related Group (DRG). The DRG associates the patient's admission with a list of specific diseases or medical conditions that require a characteristic set of tests and treatment plans and specify costs for that admission and length of stay. You will recall from previous chapters that each DRG is assumed to generate a specific amount of revenue (reimbursement) for the hospital. It is this fixed amount of money that the hospital receives no matter what tests, treatment plans, and other services are provided. If the cost of the patient's care goes above this level of reimbursement, the hospital loses money on that admission (Fig. 6-6). If the patient's care requires less services and resources, the hospital makes money on the admission. Adjustments in reimbursement for an admission that becomes more complicated than the admitting DRG are possible; however, these outliers are scrutinized very carefully by the payer.

BALANCING COST REDUCTION WITH QUALITY OF CARE

Clearly, quality of care must play a significant role under the prospective payment system and especially under capitated payment agreements. There is now a strong incentive for hospitals and physicians to reduce costs per admission by reducing the number of tests

QUALITY MANAGEMENT PLAN

▶ **FIGURE 6–7** Table of contents that shows the complexity of a hospital's quality management plan.

▶ **FIGURE 6–7** *(Continued)*

and procedures a patient receives. This can be accomplished in a few distinct ways. First, the hospital may discharge patients sooner. This allows the hospital to admit other patients sooner than expected. If this frequency continues throughout the year, more admission and DRG revenues are received. Second, the hospital can save money by reducing the number of diagnostic services for the patient by implementing shorter admission stays. Other, less obvious cost-saving efforts may be applied, including the use of alternate supplies and testing equipment or other items that do not have the capability to perform functions that may otherwise have been available.

If cost-cutting efforts are carried to the extreme, serious patient care issues could result. To counter this, the many individual CQI programs are working strenuously to define appropriate patient care standards. In addition, there is a strong and deeply rooted philosophy held by all levels of health care providers, practitioners, technologists, and nurses that patient safety and general well-being will not be compromised. In the author's experience, based on operations and budget meetings with physicians, hospital administrators, and other health care professionals, when patient safety and quality of care appear in jeopardy, decisions on behalf of the patient have been made with conviction. Also, the U.S. population has long demanded high-quality health care, and it would be surprising if this demand changed significantly. The general expectation is that public pressure will mandate that these demands continue to be met. We must also keep in mind that hospitals have a commitment to maintain appropriate health care services for the community, and CQI programs, when actively encouraged and enforced, do serve as an effective bulwark against poor quality of care.

There are other aspects of good quality care management that can save money and improve patient care. An intelligently designed and effective discharge planning program, for example, can reduce expenses by reducing patient days while providing an extremely valuable service to the patient and family. Such a cost-cutting program could include the following elements and provide important services to patients and their families:

1. Provide appropriate step-down care facilities

2. Work with insurance plans to help the patient discern among a multitude of compliance criteria regarding post-discharge care

3. Consult with patient and family to provide equipment that might be needed after discharge. Such items could include special beds, oxygen, braces, wheelchairs, etc.

4. Provide transportation between the hospital and home or to the new facility

The mission of a hospital's quality management department is very broad-based and encompasses the need to provide high-quality health care services. When complex organizations such as hospitals must function in a complex and highly regulated industry, reaching an appropriate balance between quality and expense requires a significant effort. The items listed below represent a small set of problems that must be addressed to accomplish such a balance:

1. Develop satisfactory monitors and surveys of clinical departments

2. Provide fast turnaround times for survey results

3. Formalize comprehensive annual reports for clinical departments

4. Participate in periodic quality management meetings with clinical departments

5. Assist the clinical departments in developing a regimen of service indicators

6. Assist departments in developing action plans and implementing programs of continuous quality assessment and improvement

7. Participate in team/multidisciplinary meetings during which solutions to difficult problems must be worked out to achieve the levels of effectiveness, efficiency, and appropriateness of care required

To support these activities, a detailed and comprehensive program must be developed by the hospital's quality assurance department. The author reviewed one such program. Despite the fact that the program document is written well and condensed in outline form, it is over 30 pages long. The table of contents of this document is presented in Figure 6-7 to illustrate the scope of this ongoing effort.

The amount of work, commitment, and, in some cases, tenacity that quality management departments must exhibit to accomplish this mission is extremely high. Considerable expertise is also required to work with *all* hospital personnel so that departmental barriers can be broken down and action plans can be defined, agreed upon, and implemented. Certainly, very strong support and enforcement from hospital administration is critical. Because the activities in a hospital's QM department are so closely related to reimbursement and physicians' practices, hospital administrators are usually more than willing to provide appropriate political and line management support and resources when needed. Pathways between departments and physicians must be developed to a greater degree than we have seen in the past. All employees, particularly those who have direct patient contact, must understand that it is critical to develop and adopt a service orientation and an outcome assessment philosophy in addition to enforcing practice protocols.

Quality of care efforts are now viewed as being more likely to lead to reduced rather than to increased operating costs. Indeed, quality assessment is no longer a standalone process because it has been shown that strong quality management efforts not only increase productivity and employee morale, but also assure the organization's financial viability in a tough, competitive market. In fact, many quality management programs now being developed are engineered specifically to yield defined financial goals by reducing operating inefficiencies. Such programs may include the following directives:

- Reduce cost of direct supplies
  - Medications
    - Use more generic drugs when possible
    - Use protocols that help assure that only the most effective medications are being ordered
  - Syringes, IV kits, X-ray film, IV solutions, etc.
    - Look for group purchases
    - Write longer-term purchase contracts including greater discounting with guaranteed pricing
    - Evaluate the most expensive supplies used by the department
- Reduce average length of stay
  - Develop critical paths
  - Improve discharge planning
  - Reduce days lost because patients are waiting unnecessarily for diagnostic tests
  - Develop process improvement plans
- Reduce personnel expenses
  - Reduce overtime
  - Increase cross-training where possible
- Utilization
  - Reduce number of unnecessary tests after routine hours

Surely, these cost-reduction efforts have the potential to improve patient care by reducing delays, and encouraging the use of more appropriate supplies the ordering of the most appropriate tests and medications. Such efforts and goals must be developed both at the hospital level and in each department.

QUALITY MANAGEMENT AND CQI PROGRAMS IN RADIOLOGY DEPARTMENTS

You are encouraged to locate and review a copy of the JCAHO standards and to discuss them in class. As you read through this document, it will become apparent that their primary interest is outcome-based. It is every department's responsibility to define specific methods to demonstrate that appropriate CQI efforts are ongoing.

Overseeing one of the most complex departments in the hospital, radiology directors must work toward developing well-designed and effectively implemented CQI programs. In effect, the department's CQI program can be very similar in structure to the hospital's program. The fundamental elements of a well-developed CQI program are:

1. Identify all customers for each service provided
2. The department should have a vision statement, operational goals, and clearly delineated standards for performance

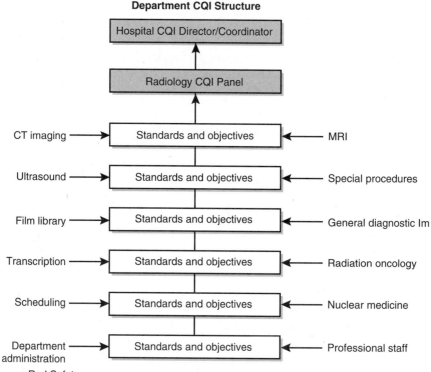

A

▶ **FIGURE 6–8** (A) Illustrates the basic structure of one radiology CQI program. (B) Identifies basic responsibilities of a department's CQI panel and mission statement. (C) An important part of a CQI program is to identify and develop a strong service orientation to its customers. The list of customers is likely to be much longer than illustrated here. (D) Shows the flow of activity that is necessary to support a department CQI program. (E) Identifies routine QA monitors that each section selects to track on an ongoing basis and documents specific focused studies for each section.

DEPARTMENT CQI PROGRAM

Mission Statement

To provide guidance, advance interest in the CQI approach, define and monitor CQI activities within the department of radiology to the extent that such efforts will cause the most effective service outcomes from individual sections as well as the aggregate service that we make available to our customers, and to develop these efforts in a fashion that is consistent with the hospital's overall quality management philosophy and its CQI programs.

Overall Responsibilities of the Department's CQI Panel

Identify customers
Develop parameters, specifications, & standards of services to customers
Report information/findings to hospital's CQI council
Work with sections to evaluate and improve services
via process improvement effort
Develops, designs, initiates, and evaluates department surveys

Monitors at least one focused study for each section per year
Monitors at least two overall department-focused studies per year

B

Identification of Customer Groups
Department of Radiology

Patients

Other hospital
departments
and nursing units

Patient relatives

Radiology services

Other nonclinical
hospital departments

Emergency department

Physicians and
their private office staff

C

▶ **FIGURE 6-8** *(Continued)*

Department of Radiology CQI Management Program
Flow Chart of Data and Activity

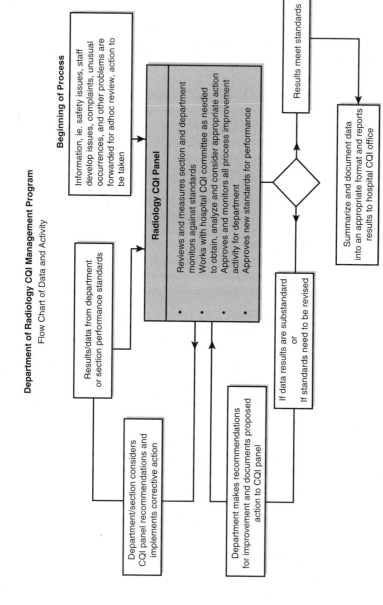

Beginning of Process

Information, ie. safety issues, staff develop issues, complaints, unusual occurrences, and other problems are forwarded for adhoc review, action to be taken

Results/data from department or section performance standards

Radiology CQI Panel

Reviews and measures section and department monitors against standards
Works with hospital CQI committee as needed to obtain, analyze and consider appropriate action
Approves and monitors all process improvement activity for department
Approves new standards for performance

Department/section considers CQI panel recommendations and implements corrective action

Department makes recommendations for improvement and documents proposed action to CQI panel

If data results are substandard or If standards need to be revised

Results meet standards

Summarize and document data into an appropriate format and reports results to hospital CQI office

D

▲ **FIGURE 6-8** *(Continued)*

Summary of Performance Indicators
and
Schedule for Review

Section _____

Year _____

Routine QC indicators	Frequency of data collection				
	Weekly	Monthly	Quarterly	Semi-Annual	Annual
1 _____					
2 _____					
3 _____					
4 _____					
5 _____					
6 _____					
7 _____					
8 _____					
9 _____					
10 _____					

Focused studies   Title of section focus studies

1 _____

2 _____

3 _____

E

▶ **FIGURE 6-8** *(Continued)*

3. A CQI panel monitoring group, or committee should be in place and composed of front-line workers rather than supervisors or managers

4. The chairperson should have management-level authority but function more as a facilitator than as an authority figure (care is necessary in selecting this person)

5. Physician involvement is vital

6. Specific reporting lines to the hospital quality management department should be defined and maintained. Some department programs include a chair on the panel for a representative from the hospital QM department

OVERVIEW OF A DEPARTMENT-BASED CQI PROGRAM

Clearly, there is no specific format that a CQI program must follow. However, the scope and nature of specific CQI initiatives are often similar among hospitals. What is important and should not vary is the commitment of the department director and the chairperson to developing an effective and ongoing program that not only measures current key services, but also continually improves current performance. Here is where these programs usually have the most difficulty. The reasons for this range from not seeing the benefit of such a comprehensive plan to poor relationships or politics within the department to a lack of vision, skill, or experience in managing these programs. A manager with relatively little experience can get valuable encouragement and help from hospital administration as well as recognition for taking the initiative to develop a strong department-based program. An experienced manager will have the confidence to target areas for improvement and to establish incentives to encourage new quality improvement efforts.

An overview of one radiology department CQI program is presented in Figure 6-8 and can be used as a model. Numerous articles and books have been written on CQI. The AHA and the American Health Care Radiology Administrators can provide a bibliography of articles and books on the topic.

S T U D Y   Q U E S T I O N S

1. Give two examples of why hospital-based quality programs have a profound effect on the overall service an institution can provide, and give two brief explanations of your examples.

2. To what degree do you think most hospitals would implement and maintain CQI programs if regulatory agencies were not in place to enforce them? Give specific examples.

3. What is the greatest change in focus that the JCAHO has taken over the past few years regarding how it measures hospital services and patient care?

4. Explain what you think the major differences are between quality assurance programs of the past and CQI programs being implemented today.

5. Using diagrams or flowcharts, develop a pictorial representation of a hospital- or department-based CQI program that you would like to implement.

6. Where does the JCAHO get its authority to credential hospitals, and who funds its operation?

7. Briefly explain the value you see in a peer review program.

8. List five of the most important elements that you believe should be in a hospital or department CQI program.

9. How do you think most physicians actually view peer review programs? Give two examples of how you think peer review has changed what they do as managers of their patients' health care needs.

SEVEN

Introduction to Radiology Department Management

OBJECTIVES FOR STUDY

After reading this chapter, the student will

▶ Appreciate the complexities of providing services and activities that are characteristic of radiology departments.

▶ Understand the interrelationships and pressures each section in radiology must handle to provide a complete radiology service.

▶ Appreciate the working environment in community, tertiary, and university hospitals.

▶ Be able to discuss the various elements that affect radiology department efficiency.

▶ Appreciate the origin of radiology services in hospitals.

▶ Understand the responsibilities of department directors and the chairperson, and the relationships between key department personnel and hospital management.

INTRODUCTION

The administrative function of radiology departments has evolved tremendously over the last 20 years to meet the increasingly sophisticated and complex demands of the health care industry. These demands have been stoked by an everchanging economic environment, which has increased the expectations of regulatory agencies, physicians, and patients. One of the most important of these expectations is that the patient, not policies or procedures, must be at the center of service. The degree to which this fundamental idea is observed within any department will determine how that department will function. Until recently, providing patients with convenient services was sometimes secondary to department processes. We are now beginning to find ways to answer fundamental patient needs without sacrificing important department processes. There is an irony in the timing of this maturation toward patient-focused care: It is not easy to provide amenities, conveniences, and flexibility of service, for example, when the importance of maximizing utilization is paramount and particularly when the availability of financial resources are as threatened as they are today in the health care industry. Such amenities and conveniences would have been much easier to implement during the better economic times of the past.

A question worthy of consideration, therefore, is how do we know when we have reached a point at which quality, utilization, and fulfilling patient expectations are in balance with reasonable cost? In short, what is optimal or appropriate care, and who will define appropriate cost?

As hospitals work to develop less and less costly operating plans, so has one of the most expensive departments in those hospitals, Radiology.

In the health care industry today, cost containment efforts often butt up against efforts to improve the quality and effectiveness of service. Because of this tension, the operational procedures and philosophies of radiology departments have come under close scrutiny, and this scrutiny has generated pressure and uncertainty among employees and caused management techniques to harden.

THE OPERATION OF RADIOLOGY DEPARTMENTS

We will attempt to provide in this chapter an inside look at the fundamental function of and work accomplished in a radiology department. We will also discuss in the next three chapters more effective ways to improve services and minimize operating costs. Not only

▶ TABLE 7–1
EMPLOYMENT OF RADIOLOGIC TECHNOLOGISTS

YEAR	TOTAL		MEN	WOMEN
1983	101,000		72,000	29,000
1988	133,000		32,000	101,000
1991	140,000		36,000	104,000
1994	154,000		39,786	114,214
Average Weekly Pay	1992	$543.00	($28,236)	
	1994	$569.00	($29,602)	

Source: U.S. Department of Labor, Bureau of Labor Statistics, 1994 tabulations.

are radiology departments among the most expensive hospital departments to operate, but also they are one of the most complex and difficult to manage. The list of high volume and widely varied activities below provides a cross section of some of the more important aspects that contribute to this complexity. The work environment of the radiology department imposes a wide range of expectations held by many different people inside and outside the hospital. This diversity of expectations narrows the acceptable margin of errors.

- Managing high-volume patient activity on a daily basis
- Managing patient transport and coordination of exams within the various sections of the department
- Monitoring patient condition and status
- Continual use, monitoring, and maintenance of complex diagnostic equipment
- Working in a highly regulated radiation environment
- Providing quality documents in picture format, which demands an understanding of technical factors and the management of multiple patient variables
- Maintaining a high volume of medical records in the form of diagnostic images and making them available to physicians and patients on demand.
- Scheduling and performing an extremely wide range of exams in conjunction with both department and referring physicians.
- Keeping the technical staff sufficiently trained with respect to new procedures and new equipment.
- Coordinating efforts with expectations of medical staff and radiologists.

THE ADMINISTRATIVE AND MANAGEMENT STRUCTURE

There are several titles associated with the position of radiology department director, so we will use the title director throughout this text for the sake of consistency. Supervisory-level duties within a department usually involve hands-on work as well as direct supervision of other employees. In larger departments, some sections (for example, the film library) are so large that an intermediate layer of managers may manage the supervisors within each section or group of sections. In other structures, one manager may be responsible for supervisors from more than one section. The two job descriptions shown in Figures 7-1 and 7-2 will clarify the difference in the scope of the director's, the managers', and the supervisors' duties. In many departments, a "lead" position is also established to take responsibility for a certain group of activities within a section.

The radiology department must provide the following fundamental services to patients and referring physicians:

- Reception/scheduling
- Transcription and recent distribution
- Clinical/diagnostic procedures
- Film filing and distribution
- Consultative services (provided by department physicians)

To provide these services, radiology departments are organized into sections. In some departments, the volume of work and general activity requires a fairly large group of employees who work only in one section. In other departments, employees rotate from section

POSITION: Administrative Director

DEPARTMENT: Radiology

IMMEDIATE SUPERVISOR: Corporate Vice President or C.O.O.

APPROVED BY: _____   DATE: _____

JOB SUMMARY:

The administrative Director of Radiology manages the department toward short term and long term goals. He or she establishes policies, procedures, standards, and objectives for the provision of medical imaging and therapeutic services. The Administrative Director evaluates performance and maintains Quality Assurance according to hospital standards as well as JCAHO, NRC, and ACR standards and regulations. The Radiology Department is managed according to hospital goals and objectives which are coordinated with other departments to provide maximum level of patient care.

PRINCIPAL DUTIES and RESPONSIBILITIES:

1. Plan, organize, staff, direct, and control department activities. Develop goals and objectives, establish and implement policies and procedures for department operation in conjunction with the Hospital Continuing Quality Improvement program and the Department Quality Improvement Team. Review department performance, effect changes as needed to improve services and assure compliance with regulatory requirements. Keep Hospital Administration and Radiologists informed of department activities, needs, and problems.

2. Select, train, and orient personnel and assign department staff. Establish work schedules according to the needs of department, evaluate performances and initiate or make recommendations for personnel actions such as merit increases, promotions, and disciplinary actions. Encourage professional development of department personnel through inservice education and outside conferences. Develops and maintains job descriptions for all staff members. Resolve staff grievances. Maintains personnel records.

3. Develops and recommends department's operating budget and ensures department operates within allocated funds. Maintains department reports and records of collected statistics for administrative and regulatory purposes. Consults with administration and Radiologists concerning capital expenditures.

4. Assures delivery of quality imaging services and therapeutic services for inpatients, outpatients, and employees. Acts as educational resource and be available for consultation to medical, nursing, and administrative staff.

5. Develops and maintains quality assurance records and techniques of the department. Evaluates radiologic functions and practices and reporting and record keeping. Complete new testing procedures and set up proto-

▶ **FIGURE 7–1** Job description for a radiology department director.

col. Introduce and demonstrate new techniques, equipment, and research findings to staff. Ensures that the department is represented on designated hospital committees.

6. Participates in administrative staff meetings and attend other meetings as required. Functions as liaison between physicians and Radiology personnel. Establishes and maintains communication within the department and with other hospital departments.
7. Develops relationships with professional affiliations and others as is appropriate.
8. Maintains department facilities and equipment and materials in a condition to promote efficiency, health, comfort, and safety of patients and staff. Assures proper storage of materials. Evaluates and justifies equipment and supply needs and purchases, negotiates, and documents maintenance schedules. Plan for use of space, purchasing new equipment, etc.
9. Establishes and maintains safety, infection, and environmental control policies and procedures for the department in cooperation with hospitalwide Safety and Infection Control committees.
10. Develops and maintains patient records within the department according to State, Federal, and regulatory agencies standards.
11. Performs duties as staff according to the needs of the department.
12. Maintains professional growth and development. Maintains professional membership in a Radiologic Technology Society.
13. Others duties as assigned according to the needs of the department.

KNOWLEDGE/SKILLS/EXPERIENCE

The Administrative Director of Radiology must have satisfactorily completed formal training in an AMA approved school of Radiologic Technology and be registered by the American Registry of Radiologic Technologists, as well as a Bachelor Degree in a business related field, with three (3) to five (5) years of supervisory experience. A Master's Degree is preferred. He or she must maintain professional growth and development to keep abreast of all functions of the Radiology Department. Participation in a professional organization, such as the American Healthcare Radiology Administrators, is encouraged.

▶ **FIGURE 7–1** *(Continued)*

POSITION: Supervisor, Film Library

DEPARTMENT: Radiology Department

IMMEDIATE SUPERVISOR: Group Manager or Admin. Director

APPROVED BY: _____   DATE: _____

JOB SUMMARY:

Under the general supervision, the Supervisor is responsible for overseeing the maintenance of all radiographic medical records.

PRINCIPLE DUTIES AND RESPONSIBILITIES:

The following statements reflect the general duties considered necessary to describe the principle functions of the job as defined and shall not be considered as a detailed description of all work requirements that may be inherent in the job.

1. Performs compiling radiographic examinations for physician interpretation and refiling for proper medical record storage.
2. Assures the proper care of radiographs coming from and going to other institutions or physician offices.
3. Files transcribed reports appropriately and accurately in patient radiograph files.
4. Pulls radiographic files daily to assist a fluent flow of patient care. Such records made available would be for all radiology department services and referring physician offices.
5. Follows specified procedures for dispatching finished reports to designated persons for approval and signature. Follows specified procedures for dispatching finished reports to appropriate parties. Oversees the disposition of finished reports to the appropriate parties.
6. Recommends necessary changes to improve clerical function. Assists in Quality Assurance studies as needed.
7. Maintains equipment in functioning order. Efficiently reports supply needs through inventory control.
8. Maintains staff work schedule. Participates in employee selection, orientation, and continuing education. Assists in the performance evaluation process for staff film librarians.
9. Other duties assigned as deemed necessary for the ongoing services of the Radiology Department.

▶ **FIGURE 7-2** Job description for a radiology department section supervisor.

to section as the need arises. The degree to which these sections function with shared or nonshared personnel is usually dependent on the department's degree of specialization and size. As patient volume and specialization increases, it usually becomes less practical for employees to rotate among sections. In fact, these sections may function very independently. Also the degree to which certification is required by each modality impacts staff rotation. A dedicated staff is needed to develop and handle the more complex operational procedures that are unique to a high volume of work. This can be better appreciated by reviewing the organization charts presented in Figures 7-3 and 7-4, which show organization charts for one radiology department in a 300-bed hospital and another in an 800-bed hospital.

HOSPITAL MISSION AND THE CONFIGURATION OF RADIOLOGY'S FLOOR PLAN

A brief review of the floor plan in Figure 7-5 will show the spatial relationship of other sections (service areas) in two very different facilities. One can clearly see how the department responsibilities of management positions can be affected by department size and by the spatial relationships sections have within a department. In addition to size and floor plan, the hospitals' mission also affects the activities and structure of the radiology department. A university-based hospital has different characteristics from a community hospital or even from a tertiary-care facility of similar size.

University-based departments are generally more complex than are community or tertiary-care facilities. There are two important reasons for this. The first is the need to engage in medical research and, more specifically, the need to infuse emerging research programs into clinical applications. Second, the presence of large numbers of medical students and residents at university based or affiliated facilities help alter the function, character, and dynamics of these departments. Some sections, like the film library, are particularly affected by this presence.

At the hospital level, a university and medical school increases management complexity by adding another layer of senior administrators over what already exists in the hospital administrative group. This can complicate the operational and financial aspects of a department significantly because the additional management layer usually leads to more political maneuvering, which often extends the decision-making process, especially when new projects are involved. In some instances, it fosters creative circumventions to obtain equipment, space, personnel, and/or services that in a less political environment could be rolled more directly and perhaps effectively into the department's operations. This is mostly felt in budget allocations.

RADIOLOGY DEPARTMENTS IN VARIOUS SETTINGS

Scope and Function of Departments

We must be careful not to confuse hospital size and the scope of radiology services a department provides with the quality of patient care. Not all large university and tertiary facilities employ cumbersome management decision-making processes nor are they less sensitive to patient needs. Similarly, not all community hospitals shortchange the public in regard to the level of expertise offered. We will define quality of care for the purpose of this discussion as the level of care a patient receives that yields positive and effective outcomes from the service provided. With this in mind, we will take a few moments to describe briefly the various types of hospitals and their departments.

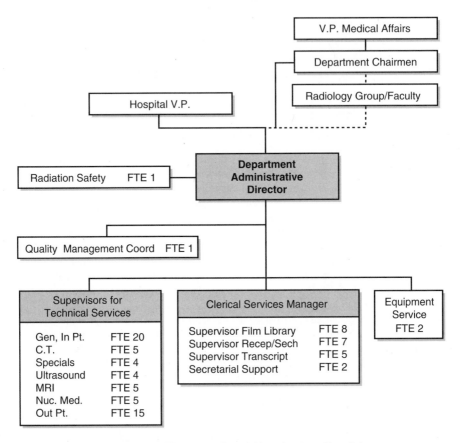

Department of Radiology Organizational Chart
300 Bed Hospital
Community or Tertiary Care

Variances in FTEs can be substantial based on type of hospital
and scope of services provided

▶ **FIGURE 7–3** An organization chart of a radiology department at a tertiary-care or community hospital.

The Community Hospital

Community hospitals are often located in suburban and rural areas and generally provide basic radiology services. Outpatient volume is generally about 60%–70%, and the payer mix and degree of discounting (collection rate) are usually dependent on the economic environment of the specific area. The atmosphere is sometimes less intense in community hospitals than in larger tertiary-care and university-based radiology departments, which may perform up to 300,000 exams per year. From the perspective of a radiology employee, workload sharing and diversity of duties are the keys to a successful community department. A typical hospital having up to approximately 300 beds will perform approximately 100,000

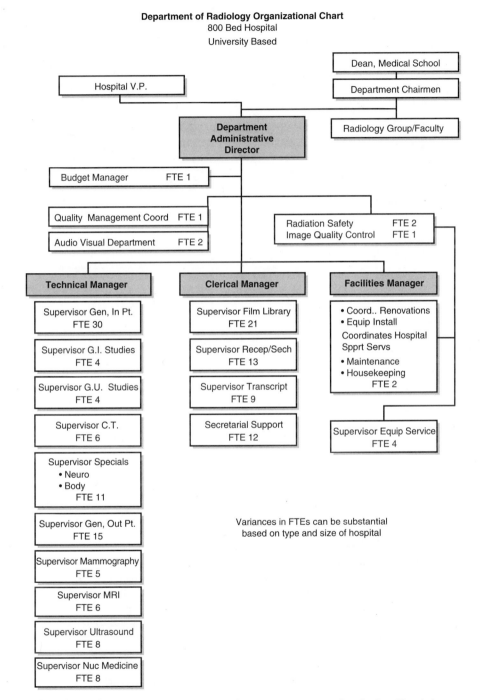

▶ **FIGURE 7-4** An organization chart of a radiology department at a university-based hospital.

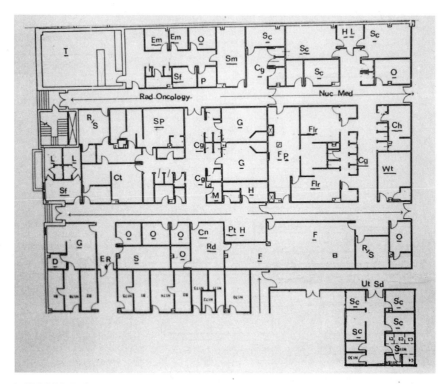

▶ **FIGURE 7–5** Floor plan of a radiology department at a 300-bed hospital with approximately 65% of its volume coming from outpatient referrals. Key: R/S, Reception scheduling; G, General radiographic rm; Flr, Fluoro rm; F, File rm; Wt, Outpt waiting; O, Office; Ch, Chest rm; Sc, Scanning rm; Sm, Treatment simulator; Sf, Lounge; Cg, Pt changing; SP, Special procedure; Em, Pt exam rm; D, Darkroom; CT, CT scanning; H, Head rm; Cn, Consultation; Rd, Reading rm; FP, Film processing; T, Treatment planning; L, Lockers; S, Storage; T, Rad. treatment.

exams per year. The department's medical staff usually functions as a private practice. The chairman of radiology usually has accountability to the hospital's vice president of medical affairs.

The Tertiary-Care Hospital

Tertiary-care hospitals evolved from community hospitals. These facilities grew rapidly as the institution's mission was altered to reach for expanded programs that provided procedures and services of increased complexity. In many instances, highly developed tertiary-care hospitals offer services similar if not identical to those offered by university-based facilities. The missing element is the degree of academic environment and commitment and drive to engage in research. The volume and complexity of clinical services provided by many tertiary-care facilities are similar to those provided by university-based hospitals. In fact, many of the tertiary-care facilities the author has visited could serve as operational models for efficiency and effectiveness in regards to patient services. Tertiary-care facilities usually have from 400 to 800 beds and have highly trained and competent technical and medical staffs.

University-Based Hospitals

What separates university-based hospitals from other hospitals is their academic atmosphere, which encourages medical research, publishing, and lecturing and the constant pursuit of research grants from federal, state, and private organizations. Reputation is a key driving force in all university-based hospitals because an institution's reputation is important in part in the competition for grant money. Grants can bring millions of dollars annually into a department to support research activities. In fact, in some departments, research efforts seem to permeate almost every element of operation: It is not unusual for a department to have from $10 to $30 million dollars in research grants supporting its various programs at any given time.

A high reputation also brings prominent physicians to the faculty, who in turn design research projects that win more grants. This reputation also helps to generate new patient referrals as new and emerging clinical techniques and procedures are used to treat advanced, complex, and rare diseases. For awhile, one university-based hospital's marketing slogan was "Our doctors write the papers other doctors read." The emphasis of this marketing effort was to establish a sense of leadership in research and medical knowledge.

Although research is very significant to the advancement of medical care, the manner in which this knowledge is applied at university-based hospitals is sometimes criticized, primarily for leading to a lack of a patient-friendly environment. University-based medical centers frequently consist of a matrix of buildings and abound with medical students and residents. This cadre of physicians sometimes confuses patients who want to know who their physician actually is.

SPECIALIZATION AMONG RADIOLOGISTS

In some community hospital departments, radiologists rotate fairly equally to perform almost all procedures. In university-based hospitals, radiologists specialize their interest to a specific body region or body function. Depending on the size of the facility, the degree of specialization can range from moderate to high. At the far end of the specialization spectrum, we find that university-based radiologists often develop a fairly circumscribed set of clinical skills and perform tests and procedures that are unique to its subspecialty. Such specialization is indicated by the organization charts and floor plans shown earlier. The GI section, for example, operates as an area separate and distinct from the bone section or the CT section within radiology. Also often, each section has its own technical supervisor and chief radiologist, who is commonly referred to as the section chief. In each of these sections, the section chief has full professor status with the medical school and is responsible for the medical care provided in the specialty or section. He or she is also principally responsible for teaching medical students and residents his or her unique skills in that specialty. Each of these sections often has a dedicated and highly skilled technical staff as well.

The technical supervisor and the section chief share responsibility for running their area. They set their work schedules under general department guidelines and develop their own operational policies, which must, however, be in concert with those approved by the department director and chairperson.

Such a department may have as many as 12 distinct clinical sections, which in aggregate perform up to approximately 800 to 900 exams each weekday. In this high-volume and highly specialized environment, staff radiologists do not rotate through other sections. However, radiology residents do rotate among the different services and acquire a well-rounded training experience. Operationally and managerially, this degree of subspecialization can cause inefficiencies, but it is ideal for training residents, who get the benefit of working with some of the most specialized and skilled faculty in the world in a particular subspecialty of radiology. Also, patients receive the benefit of having their tests performed or at least reviewed by the most highly regarded physicians in the county or world in that specialty.

OPERATIONAL CHARACTERISTICS

Regardless of their size or scope of service, radiology departments generate a wide variety of internal operational challenges. For instance, one of the principal difficulties in operating a large department is that each section (e.g., film library, reception, and the various clinical sections) will want and often need to function as a unique operation with unique policies and procedures that are designed to regulate its activities. As these sections grow and change, it is important for the department to keep them in phase with other sections and to review performance indicators that measure effectiveness continuously.

We must be mindful of the difference between effectiveness and efficiency. A highly efficient section may not necessarily be highly effective. Such a section may accomplish its many internal tasks and jobs with precision, yet the section's overall effectiveness may be lacking in its ability to serve those outside the section. For example, some of these duties, jobs, or procedures may be too self-focused and not contribute significantly to patient care or to the overall service that is expected of the department. It is important to realize that almost every one of these discrete section duties should have some effect on the overall service of the department. The degree to which this occurs indicates the section's effectiveness. It is also possible for several sections to be operating efficiently within themselves but not to be in synch with the other sections of the department. It is the director's responsibility to be mindful of this and to monitor continuously these aspects of the department to make sure that section activities are integrated and support the radiology service overall. The degree to which integration and coordination occur will often determine the overall quality and effectiveness of the department as viewed by patients and referring physicians.

THE MANAGEMENT STRUCTURE

Figures 7-3 and 7-4 show organizational charts with full time equivalent (FTE) worker distributions against overall patient/exam volume. By reviewing these charts and statistics, one can begin to appreciate that as a department becomes more complex, its efficiency and effectiveness can be affected. However, it is not at all a given that large departments are automatically inefficient or ineffective. The author has visited many large departments that produce huge volumes of work per day. In these departments, work in each section is properly integrated with the efforts of the other sections and is in synch with the department's mission and service objectives.

OTHER ASPECTS OF DEPARTMENT EFFICIENCY AND EFFECTIVENESS

Note the elements for evaluating efficiency shown in Table 7-2. Tertiary-care and university-based hospitals rely on the availability of sophisticated high-tech services to diagnose and treat less common diseases and disorders. In order to provide these special services, the facility must attract and keep physicians who have a higher than average level of expertise or special experience in handling these conditions. In addition, such services require more specialized and often more expensive equipment. Also, highly trained and specialized personnel are needed to operate this equipment and assist these physicians. In addition to the need for very specialized equipment and personnel, a third factor affects cost—the use of more complex protocols to perform procedures and diagnostic tests. These protocols are defined by the physician in charge. This, in fact, poses a dilemma to many radiology department directors, who must work to reduce operating costs and services without diluting the quality of these studies or making the cost of these studies too high in relation to costs at other facilities. The need to balance cost against the implementation of sophisticated protocols is continually challenging department directors and requires continuous support from the department chairperson and medical and technical staff.

We have seen how highly specialized and dedicated equipment and highly skilled radiologists and technologists can add to overall operating costs. Department directors and chairpersons thus feel continuous pressure from hospital administrations to reduce operating costs across the entire department and to look for cost-effective alternatives that will not diminish service. Thus, the challenge is to bring the factors listed below into balance:

- Availability and convenience of service to patients and referring physicians
- Quality of service and care
- Cost
- Scope and complexity of services provided

▶ TABLE 7−2
COMMONLY USED DEPARTMENT PRODUCTIVITY MEASUREMENTS

ANNUAL CALCULATIONS
Number of radiology exams performed
Number of inpatient exams performed
Number of outpatient exams performed
Number of hospital admissions
Number of patients seen in the ED
Number of patients referred by ED
Number of portables/OR exams performed
Number of stat portable exams performed
Number of technologists per outpatient exams performed
Number of technologists per inpatient exams performed
Number of technologists per total exams performed
Number of technologists per staffed bed
Number of nontechnical FTEs per staffed bed
Number of inpatient exams per admission (differentiate amb. care & ED)
Number of RVUs generated
Number or RVUs generated by a specific work area or section
Number of technologists per RVU for specific technical area or section
Number of nontechnical staff per RVU for each work area
Number of portable studies per staffed bed

Common elements used to help measure and define productivity of radiology department personnel and equipment.

Just like departments in tertiary-care and university-based settings, departments in community hospitals are also experiencing serious cost-reduction pressures aimed at improving the efficiency and effectiveness of services offered. Department directors in these facilities must find ways to build more flexibility into staffing assignments and duties. When vacancies occur, it may be necessary to continue for an extended time with such vacancies rather than immediately to fill them. Yet, with fewer people on staff, the flexibility needed to train and rotate personnel is reduced. Despite these difficulties, it is necessary to have each staff member cover a broader range of duties as vacancies occur. The need to encourage cross-training has indeed increased over recent years.

SETTING OPERATIONAL STANDARDS

The need to define operational goals and expectations is universal throughout the health care industry. Over the last 30 years, certain major industries have gone through tremendous economic stress and organizational shake-ups. In the 1960s, it was the automotive industry that was in trouble; in the 1970s, it was the steel industry; and in the 1980s, the banking industry came close to collapse. In each of these cases, a lack of efficient and effective operating procedures and poor financial management led to financial turbulence. In the 1990s, it is the health care industry that faces new demands for more services as pressure to reform its entire delivery system increases to a degree not seen in the history of medicine.

The health care industry's ability to meet the challenges of a cost-driven environment without jeopardizing the underpinnings of a system that provides access to the highest-skilled medical professionals in the world is being tested to an unprecedented degree. Knowing when to stop cutting expenses, not just how to cut them, is of primary importance. One approach that can be used to help define necessary services and expenses lies in defining fairly specific standards and objectives for performance and service and, in doing so, to identify *specific customers* who will be served by those standards. Such operational standards become specifications for performance and ideally should be developed for each section within a department. Figure 7-6 shows a brief outline of an operational program that was developed for a particular section within a radiology department. Such specifications of operations also help to define staffing needs and supply costs.

MEASUREMENTS OF DEPARTMENT EFFICIENCY

Operational standards and goals should not be used without some measure of comparison with peer facilities. It is the responsibility of department management to compare current operational standards continuously with those of other facilities that offer similar ranges of services and handle similar patient volume. Although comparison summaries can be helpful in evaluating one's own service, we must understand that even the most controlled survey can yield data that are meaningless and out of context. Therefore, all survey data must be scrutinized to the degree that outliers are accounted for and understood.

An example of such an outlier may be that department A's total FTE count is considerably lower than that of department B. This may be because department A's patient transport or escort workers are assigned to the hospital's central escort pool. In another example, department A's reception/scheduler FTE count may be higher than that of department B. This may be because hospital A's receptionists are required to take patients' insurance information and apply reimbursement codes in addition to scheduling and receiving patients. Such questions must be asked before any survey can be taken seriously. If serious discrepancies

---

OPERATIONS PLAN

I. Definition of mission
II. Definition of specific goals & objectives
III. Definition of key positions & their principal responsibilities
IV. Hours of operation
V. Definition of whom service is aimed at
VI. Definition of productivity standards
VII. Key indicators that will be used to measure outcome/success of service

---

▶ **FIGURE 7-6** Outline of an operating plan for a radiology department or section.

arise, one may talk with the principal investigator/coordinator of the survey in an effort to get more detailed background information.

Administrators at more and more hospitals are using this type of comparative data and to encourage department directors to define new productivity standards. It is important for radiology management to understand how this information can be used appropriately and effectively so that efficiency can be improved without sacrificing basic quality of service. There are several groups or organizations that collect and provide productivity reports. Many university hospitals, for example, belong to an organization called the University Hospital Consortium. This organization has many functions, including establishing large multihospital group purchasing agreements which have the potential to yield high discounts on a wide variety of supplies and major equipment purchases. Many other hospitals belong to the Volunteer Hospital Association (VHA). Services provided by the VHA are very broad in scope and include the development and management not only of traditional group purchasing agreements, but also in some instances management services. In the end, however, it is the department director's role to define what an acceptable level of efficiency is for his or her department and how this benchmark can be appropriately translated into an effective service. From a more general perspective, a given department's efficiency, as shown previously, is to a large degree dependent on the aggregate of the various department characteristics and attributes shown below. One should also keep in mind the list of elements that cause the high level of complexity that was discussed earlier in this chapter.

1. A well- and appropriately developed department management structure

2. A well-developed organization chart that is understood by all department employees

3. Staffing adequate to provide required services and to meet fundamental expectations of all customers the department serves

4. A department floor plan that adequately provides for the logistical needs of patient services, employees' communication needs, and basic environmental needs (such as air conditioning; phone lines; clean, wide corridors through which patients and equipment can be moved)

5. A clear understanding of appropriately defined department and section service objectives not only by management but also by all employees

6. A clear understanding of department operational expectations by sections within the department and customers outside the department

7. A clear understanding of the products each section produces and who the customers are who depend on the department to provide those products

Responsibilities of the Department Director

As we have seen from the job descriptions presented in Figures 7-1 and 7-2, department directors must assume general responsibility for all the various elements below:

- Efficiency of the service
- Personnel competence
- Morale
- Image quality
- Finances
- Equipment acquisition and maintenance
- Maintenance of appropriate records and documents
- Provision of functions that are in concert with the various regulatory agencies
- Minimization of cost
- Utilization of personnel, floor space, and equipment
- Services that are integrated with other hospital departments

This matrix of responsibilities often creates conflict, in the sense that maintaining effective operations is dependent upon a well-trained and content staff. Continuous pressures to shrink budgets can sometimes generate hidden costs and work against efforts to keep staff morale high. Sometimes the less-defined requirements in the department director's job description are more vital to the service offered the customer than are the requirements that have been written. For example, it is essential for the department director to communicate effectively with hospital administration, the medical staff, and department personnel. It is also essential that new perspectives on difficult issues are considered thoroughly and implemented effectively. Further, it is essential that the director develop and maintain a high professional profile for the department. Integrity, trust, competence, experience, and a general sense of decency are among the most vital attributes a person needs to fill this role successfully.

The department director must interact effectively with key people on the department's medical staff. Coordination between the section supervisor, the section chief, the managers, and the chairperson as well as other section managers (such as those in the file room, scheduling, and reception) can become challenging. It is also important for the department director to have freedom to make decisions and changes without unnecessary intervention from the chairperson.

THE ROLE OF SECTION SUPERVISORS AND MANAGERS

Supervisory and management personnel are also demanding positions. Their responsibility is to work hand-in-hand with the people they supervise while attending to a growing list of administrative demands and requirements. They are on the front lines with their employees but at the same time must maintain the difficult posture of keeping a certain distance and objectivity so management decisions can be made and executed fairly. Being able to handle the pressures of this bimodal responsibility consistently can be extremely challenging. For these reasons, successful supervisors are highly regarded employees. Their efforts in supervising a section so that it performs consistently well and effectively supports the department's mission and operational objectives deserve high recognition.

THE DEPARTMENT CHAIRPERSON AND HOSPITAL ADMINISTRATION

The degree to which the chairperson and radiologists become involved in making operational decisions in a department varies considerably from one department to another. There is no clear pattern concerning how much direct management influence the chairperson will have. However, there is considerable evidence that hospital administrations view the radiology director's role as an extension of hospital administration rather than as an extension of the chairperson's position. This separation of management from medical affairs at the department level is evolving rapidly as some hospital administrators feel mounting pressure to cut operating costs and to integrate radiology services with other hospital-based services to a greater degree. Still other hospital administrators see the management and medical practice as a necessary synergy. In this model line responsibility includes the chairperson.

Separation of responsibilities between the chairperson and the director has the potential to cause increased conflict, however. Despite this potential, the relationship between the department director and the chief radiologist or chairperson is very important and must be based on trust and a spirit of collaboration because it is virtually impossible to separate the specific medical practice of radiology from the management and operational decisions made to support patient care services. This relationship is also important to understand because in many instances, the work habits of the radiology group and the chairperson can affect personnel decisions. Personnel decisions are integral to defining the department's organization chart and to selecting supervisors and managers. To the department director, having the freedom to make these decisions is as important to the success of any policy or operations process as it is to the success of the chairperson's decisions about his or her section chiefs or associates.

REPORTING LINES OF THE RADIOLOGY DIRECTOR

The director must be free to make decisions that may not be popular and that may affect the practicing patterns of the department. The department director in many cases has a dual responsibility: Although he or she must work with the chairperson and individual members of the radiology group, the director often has *line responsibility,* or reports directly to the VP at the hospital level. This dual responsibility has the potential to generate conflict because the department chairperson and the hospital VP may not share the same goals, or at least the same priorities. This, of course, can lead to serious problems.

Communication between radiology and hospital administration is especially vital when there is disagreement concerning goals or priorities between the chairperson and the VP. Under these circumstances, the department director is sometimesviewed as the principal liaison between the hospital administration, radiologists, and, when necessary, other employees.

A BRIEF HISTORY OF HOSPITAL-BASED RADIOLOGY SERVICES

A brief history regarding the evolution of radiology services can lead to a better understanding of the current state of the department of radiology. X rays were described by Wilhelm Conrad Roentgen (1845–1923), a German physicist, while he was working with vacuum tubes operating at high voltages. When an electrical current passed between the positively and negatively charged points of the tube in a dark room, it excited a supply of platinocyanide which had been casually stored nearby. Roentgen concluded that the voltage moving through the vacuum tube must have emitted an energy form that was unknown. This new energy, Roentgen deduced, was transmitted from the tube and caused a reaction within the platinocyanide that was sufficient to induce the glow he had observed. After his discovery on November 8, 1895, Roentgen published papers describing this phenomenon which carried the news around the world. As early as on January 2, 1896, Michael Idvorsky Pupin, a professor at Columbia University, produced the first known radiographic image in the United States. Such experiments soon occurred routinely, and this research quickly took on additional momentum as new tubes and light emitting materials (phosphorescents) were discovered. Thomas Edison experimented with calcium tungstate, which he showed to have better emission properties. This led to Edison's development of the earliest fluoroscopy devices. Indeed, the disciplines of basic science and medicine had been inexorably coupled to produce what would become one of the most dynamic and beneficial medical specialties yet developed.

The earliest radiology departments began to take form during the late 1800s. They were established as one-room operations, and physicians in many instances volunteered their time to work with the new investigative tool of X-radiation. The interest in producing and interpreting roentgenograms, as they were often called, for medical purposes grew rapidly as a number of publications advanced the value they had in medical science. The desire to develop a science of image production and interpretation among these volunteer X-ray physicians eventually forced the emergence of a more defined service. The rate at which this evolution occurred in each hospital was significantly affected by the number of patients sent to have this new diagnostic test and the investigative drive of the medical staff. As the degree of dependency on diagnostic X-ray imaging increased, these fledgling roentgenologists reached a point at which they either had to dedicate the balance of their medical careers to radiology or had to return to their previous practices.

The physicians who elected to continue their careers in radiology had to discuss facility and compensation issues with hospital administrations. It should be kept in mind that, at that time, hospital administrations often consisted of one full-time superintendent or manager. How much space could and should be dedicated to radiology? How would these new services provided by the physician be valued and paid for? How would equipment be purchased? These were some of the perennial issues that required resolution. As a result of these discussions, significant differences in priorities and philosophies between the administrators and roentgenologists began to emerge, but in the end, agreements were eventually negotiated and signed. Some of these agreements allowed the radiologist to purchase the equipment and to hire and pay his or her people. In return for the use of hospital space, the radiologist would pay rent to the hospital. In this case, the radiologist would collect all revenue for the services provided. In effect, a radiology concession was formed. Hospital administrators benefitted by such a contract because they were assured of a service for their patients without taking on the added worry related to personnel management, equipment acquisition, and operating expenses for a new science they knew little or nothing about. At the other extreme, contracts were also written whereby the radiologist became salaried and agreed to work in the hospital as a full-time employee. In this case, all equipment, personnel, and associated expenses were covered by the hospital. There were also variations on these two basic models.

At times, the advantages of having either type of contract did not seem obvious, and there was in fact debate as to who wanted these advantages. With ownership comes responsibility for cost and immediate operational worries. However, accepting the responsibility for the cost and risk of any organization eventually leads to control of that organization. Over time, the principal advantage seemed to lie in control of the service, and accepting financial and operating risks was—and still is—viewed as necessary by hospital administrations.

THE FORMALIZATION OF RADIOLOGY SERVICES

Hospitals were very interested in securing contracts with radiologists because they insured continued radiology services for their patients. Hospital administrators also wanted to have these services available to the physicians on their medical staffs. The demand for radiology services and advances in its technology accelerated by 1910. In addition, the prestige associated with offering these services brought increased recognition to facilities, which in turn could attract more physicians to join their staffs. Other hospital physicians also encouraged contracts with radiologists in order to gain assurance that this new diagnostic tool would be at their disposal.

Interest in diagnostic radiology began to grow more and more rapidly as new equipment and imaging techniques were introduced through the 1920s. Never before had a new science and its associated hardware been so closely linked to medicine. Electrical engineers and physicists worked closely with physicians to design and manufacture equipment. It also became clear that the cost of this new service would be great. This cycle of research and clinical application leading inevitably to new and growing demands for services and more research brought about a rapid expansion of capabilities and costs, a cycle that is still in place today. However, these new services in turn generated new patient referrals and revenue. Soon, larger dedicated areas for radiology services and additional medical staff had to be provided.

OUR PROFESSION AND ITS GOVERNANCE

The principal and most central authority for certifying practicing radiology technologists is the american Registry of Radiologic Technologists. This body was born in 1920 when a small group of radiologists working out of the Radiological Society of North America and the American Roentgen Ray Society advocated certification of persons operating X-ray equipment. In 1923, the Registry was fully established and began to implement rules of operation and a charge of responsibilities.

The American Registry of Radiologic Technologists (ARRT) of today is governed by a board of trustees formed by eight members. Four are appointed by the American Society of Radiologic Technologists and four appointed by the American College of Radiology. The activities of the ARRT are supported by an executive director, a small group of assistants, and a cadre of staff people. The ARRT's major responsibility lies in defining standards for certification of all technical subspecialties dealing with radiation diagnostic imaging, including CT and MRI, and keeping track of all associated records.

Another important professional organization has its roots in the early 1900s. Ed C. Jerman brought together 13 other X-ray pioneers from across the United States and Canada to provide a central source of information and a professional body that could coordinate educational programs and distribute technical information for the benefit of its members, who perform tests in all subspecialties typically associated with radiology. This organization is known today as the American Society of Radiologic Technologists (ASRT); it was formerly known as the American Association of Radiological Technicians. The first issue of its journal, *X-Ray Technician,* was published in July 1929. Today, this journal is titled *Radiologic Technology.*

The ASRT operated through a cadre of volunteer officers and staffers who developed rules and policies of governance until 1946, when one full-time staff person was hired as executive secretary. The society developed philosophies regarding various developments that involved the profession and its members and lobbied to advocate these positions. Examples of such developments were the issues of state certification and implementation of specified curriculum for school certification by the AMA. One of its noteworthy initiatives was realized when President Reagan signed the Consumer-Patient Radiation Health Act in 1981. This established rigid standards for accreditation of educational programs for those who administer ionizing radiation.

The earliest radiology departments had emerged as fully recognized stand-alone services by 1905 (Fig. 7-7). New staffing needs also emerged as demands for larger and more complex equipment were answered. The need to train a dedicated and more skilled nonphysician work force was also becoming apparent. People who had an interest in working with this new medical science had to be hired and trained as apprentices under the direction of radiologists. As in earlier medical history, the three cities that dominated investigative testing and the clinical use of X rays for imaging were Boston, Philadelphia, and New York.

RADIOLOGY EVOLVES TOWARD A HOSPITAL-BASED SERVICE

Through the early 1900s, a variety of working agreements between hospital administrators and radiologists flourished. Until about 1950, the radiology concession was common. However, in the early 1960s, legal, operational, and personnel management issues began to cause problems for hospital administrations and their employees. Significant personnel issues regarding equity of salary and benefits between radiology employees and other hospital employees became problematic: In many instances, benefits for radiology employees were much greater. Hospital administrators were often put in compromising positions when trying to explain to nonradiology employees why Radiology had a different compensation and benefit program.

As radiology departments grew in size, their independence and political strength also increased. Many large departments had evolved into multimillion-dollar operations. Many departments employed more than 100 people. Coordinating hospital management philosophies with radiology department management philosophies often proved difficult. Labor relations practices regarding the termination of employees, personal leaves, and promotions were sometimes conducted differently in Radiology. Such issues began to draw unavoidable attention from hospital attorneys, who were needed to settle employee claims of unfair labor practices. Stronger federal laws regarding labor issues enacted during this time also increased hospital administrators' concerns.

Other issues began to emerge as well. Beginning in the 1950s, non-Radiology physicians began to acquire X-ray equipment to be used and installed their own services. In some instances, this created duplication of equipment and created the potential for turf wars regarding which service—for example, Orthopedics or Radiology—would be allowed to operate X-ray equipment. Such turf wars encourage political maneuvering, confusion, and

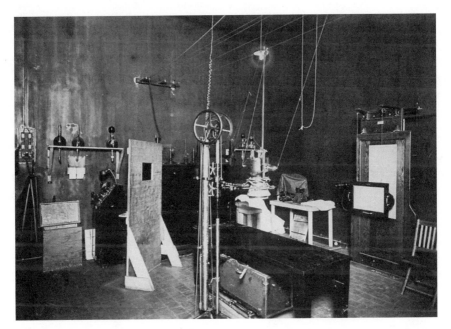

▶ **FIGURE 7-7** Shows the type of equipment utilized in facilities around 1919. (Source: The National Library of Medicine.)

disharmony in an organization. Hospital administrators frequently had to settle such disputes knowing that the chances for reaching a decision that would satisfy everyone were slim. In short, the stand-alone radiology concession created integration problems and issues of parity within the organization. The first step toward resolving these concerns was to merge radiology into the hospital's operation more effectively; hospital administrators began to move slowly in this direction. Contracts leading to control of radiology departments were negotiated much more strenuously during the 1960s. Transitions between old and new Radiology chairpersons provided hospitals with opportunities to write contracts having more and more limitations and requirements regarding the chairperson's span of control over department operations and department finances.

Today, contracts assume hospital control of financial and nonmedical operational decisions. The primary link between the hospital administration and the radiology department is through the department director. The chairperson is expected to exercise his or her effort primarily to advance new medical applications and to build a staff of highly skilled radiologists. Hospitals continue to depend on the chairperson to advise hospital administrators in the delivery of quality medical care. The chairperson is dependent in turn on the hospital for the basic facilities, staffing, equipment, and management services needed to provide the appropriate level of diagnostic and treatment services to referring physicians at the recommended scope of medical services needed.

Thus, a somewhat symbiotic relationship must exist between those who make the financial and management decisions and those who provide a high-quality medical service. The hospital, on the other hand, must fulfill facility needs to encourage and support continued growth of these referrals. However, under the evolving managed care capitated contracts, the chairperson and his or her staff must serve as effective advisors to the medical staff by providing direction on which tests and modalities are most likely to yield diagnostic answers to the medical condition. The effectiveness of this council helps the institution reduce operating costs and increase efficiency of hospital services as a whole, which can often translate into an earlier discharge.

The chairperson can earn considerable political strength among the general medical staff by providing a top-flight service. In many cases, this political strength has been leveraged to encourage hospitals to provide resources that otherwise may not have been granted. As hospitals experience increasing economic pressure, though, the bargaining power of most chairpersons has been substantially reduced. All departments of a hospital must compete for their shares of the hospital's financial pie. This is particularly true when capital funds are at stake. You will recall that the operating budget is influenced by the capital budget. Thus, negotiations for capital money are an extremely important activity, and are sometimes a precursor to increased operating expenses that will continue for many years into the future.

DEFINING SECTION SERVICES AND INDIVIDUAL EFFORTS

The author has used several techniques to improve services and maintain a high level of performance by each section in the radiology department. One of the most comprehensive and effective approaches is to develop a service program for each section of the department. To accomplish this, a detailed program including the following basic elements needs to be developed:

- Productivity measures
- Mission statement
- Objectives of the service
- Criteria for quantifying and measuring level and quality of service
- Support procedures/policies
- Scope of services provided

Each of these elements must be developed properly and reviewed with all supervisors in the section. The chairperson and members of the radiology group must also have an opportunity to critique and comment. Supervisors should allow their staff to do the same before the final copy is distributed. In addition, a similar program should be developed by the department director for the overall department service, which is reviewed with radiologists and the management group. This in effect becomes the operations plan for each section that supports the overall radiology program. The quality and degree of detail built into these plans will have a direct bearing on their effectiveness in improving the department service. It also helps to outline each employee's role in this effort, which establishes clear expectations for both the management team and department employees. The written program for a given section may be up to 10 pages long.

NURSING SERVICES IN RADIOLOGY

We must consider the patients basic needs and how they are monitored. Several patients with a wide variety of medical-care needs may be in the department. The logistics of scheduling patients—seeing that they arrive and leave with a minimum of waiting—is a major undertaking every day of the week and, as mentioned above, the complexity of this task is compounded by the variety of medical needs each patient may have.

An important part of this aspect of the radiology service is the nursing skills that are available. Almost all departments have full-time nursing personnel to take care of the medical needs of the patients who are waiting in the department or who are having procedures. Sometimes, department nurses are actually employees of the nursing department who have been scheduled to work in radiology. In other instances, nurses are on the department's payroll. In either case, their availability is extremely important to assure good patient care. If special procedures are performed in radiology, nurses may be needed to monitor the patient's vital signs and administer medication. They may also be needed to monitor the medical status of patients who are waiting pre- or postexam to make sure that their vital signs are stable and under control.

SUMMARY

In this chapter, we have provided an overview of radiology management and a brief sample of some of the pressures and political issues that are a part of daily operations in the radiology department. It is important for the reader to have a clear understanding of the enormous amount of planning, coordination, and preparation that is needed consistently from the director and the supervisory group to make sure that the service provided is optimal. There is no question, however, that this level of supervision would go for nought if it were not for dedicated and talented clerical and technical staff members, who must work together and with each patient. The risk of error generated by the variety and range of tasks performed throughout the day is huge. It must be the responsibility of every individual to keep these tasks as error-free as possible. All department employees must continually keep in mind that any error can jeopardize the overall effort of many employees and that these errors can affect the patient's well-being and overall quality of the service.

We have heard a great deal about focusing all this effort on the patient, and make no mistake: This is the principal reason we are here. The economic pressures to reduce operating costs while increasing and improving patient services force new priorities and alliances. The need for hospitals to win provider contracts with HMOs, Blue Cross, and PPOs is clearly a matter of survival, and it is incumbent upon each manager and each employee to provide the best effort possible to help assure that his or her facility will be sought out by managed care payers when bidding begins. In short, these efforts do represent a fundamental form of job security.

STUDY QUESTIONS

1. Define at least three aspects of the overall radiology service that contribute to its unique operational aspects.
2. What are the characteristics that distinguish departments that are located in community, tertiary-care, and university-based hospitals? Also, how might the strengths or missions of these three facilities differ?
3. The matter of efficiency has been addressed several times throughout this text. As department director, how would you define department efficiency? Give two philosophies that you believe must be in place before a high level of efficiency can be achieved.
4. Distinguish between department efficiency and effectiveness. Do you think it is possible to obtain high efficiency and yet have an ineffective service? If so, give one example.

5. Select three responsibilities that you believe are very important for a department director to assume and explain why you think they are particularly important.

6. As a supervisor of a section in Radiology, describe what your concerns might be in balancing your efforts to work with employees while satisfying operations requirements for a highly efficient and low-cost service.

Logistics and Intradepartmental Dependencies

O B J E C T I V E S F O R S T U D Y

After reading this chapter, the student will

▶ Understand the primary activities and responsibilities of each section (work area) of a radiology department and the particular aspects of those responsibilities that generate significant stress.

▶ Appreciate several features needed to provide a comprehensive and quality-oriented service to patients and referring physicians.

▶ Appreciate the concept of an organizational pecking order and how this may affect decision making at the hospital level.

▶ Understand the various personal needs each patient has regarding privacy, security, and safety.

▶ Understand the "service" aspect of working with patients and how this not only improves quality of service to the patient, but also affects the department's marketability.

INTRODUCTION

In Chapter Seven, we saw that radiology services have evolved from humble beginnings into today's sophisticated and highly dynamic medical specialty that touches almost every individual and physician in the country. We also noted the significant financial resources needed to support these services as well as the major political tensions that exist among medical staff, hospital administration, and department administration.

We also considered some of the internal issues that must be addressed in order to maintain the management and financial controls that must be in place to assure effectiveness. In this regard, we noted that all sections in Radiology must strive to perform in a coordinated fashion to provide as timely and error-free a service as possible to its patients. We will now look at each of these sections in slightly more detail to gain an insider's appreciation of the logistics that are actually involved in providing a high-quality, cost-effective, and comprehensive radiology service. We will also consider the sections' various tasks and responsibilities with a focus on the various sections' mutual dependencies.

Each section of Radiology carries out a unique set of responsibilities and services, yet each of these areas must work in close synchronization to produce a complete radiology service. Coordinating the multitude of activities in these sections is the key to success. In very large hospitals, these sections may be distributed over five or six different buildings. In fact, the overall space requirement for such a department can exceed 100,000 square feet, and there may be more than 50 procedure rooms. To gain some perspective on this, keep in mind that the playing surface of a football field is 48,000 square feet. Although it is a significant task to coordinate such a large department, it can be equally stressful to manage a department that has less patient volume and less floor space. Instead of depending on several relatively independent sections, smaller departments must build in a high degree of flexibility among its employees so they can work in more than one area of the department. For this reason, each person's effort has a greater impact on the final product. If coordination between sections and personnel is not achieved, the first person who usually feels the effect is the patient or the referring physician.

SCHEDULING AND RECEPTION SERVICES

Radiology department work begins with schedulers who schedule exams and register patients. The exam schedule is usually done over the phone. It is extremely important for several reasons that all patient demographic information is entered into a computer or paper file accurately. Keeping patients safe from unnecessary untoward effects of treatment is dependent on such seemingly small details as spelling their names correctly so that their records will not be confused with other patients' files. Many patient injuries and law suits have resulted directly or in part from patients receiving inappropriate services or procedures because their records incorrectly showed no contraindications or warnings to alert the physician or technologist in advance. In other instances, patients have received exams that were to be performed on someone else due to inaccurate documentation of patient records. Radiologists and the patient's physician may have difficulty locating complete files because they didn't know that a second or duplicate jacket exists, even though that jacket may contain important diagnostic information. This can delay the radiologists' interpretation and final reports. Worse yet, inaccurate demographic information entered into a patient's record can result in X-ray images of two different patients being labeled under one name and filed in one jacket. Figure 8-1 shows a standard radiology requisition form.

DEPARTMENT OF RADIOLOGY
EXAMINATION REQUEST

Case No. _____
New _____
Old _____
Date _____

PATIENT ACCOUNT NUMBER		ROOM AND BED NO.	MEDICAL RECORD NUMBER

PATIENT

PATIENT'S NAME AND ADDRESS.	DATE	TIME OF ARRIVAL	AGE	MS	SEX	NO INS.

ADMISSION DATE		PATIENT D.O.B.	F.C.

HOME PHONE NO.	SOCIAL SECURITY NO.	INS CO		GROUP NO.: POLICY NO.: SOC. SEC. NO.:

	CODE	SUBSCRIBER	REL

INSURANCE

GUARANTOR NAME AND ADDRESS	REL	INS CO		GROUP NO.: POLICY NO.: SOC. SEC. NO.:

	CODE	SUBSCRIBER	REL

EMPLOYER NAME AND ADDRESS	M/S	CODE	MED. CLAIM NO.	PTA(H)	PTB(M)	SUBSCRIBER

MA	CODE	CD	RECORD NO.	CAT	CO	LN #	RES	EXPIRE DATE

PRIORITY: ORDERED: CONTROL #:

PORTABLE: TRANSPORT: ORDER DOCTOR:

PART TO BE EXAMINED:

REASON FOR EXAM:

PREGNANT: ALLERGIES: LAST MENSTRUAL PERIOD:

COMMENTS:

▶ **FIGURE 8–1** Shows a typical requisition form for obtaining an imaging study. This is a legal document that can carry important information provided by several different services. This document should be respected for the clinical information it contains and because it is used in the courts to help determine liability.

The complexity of scheduling exams is actually much greater than may appear at first. Schedulers deserve a great deal of credit for the effort and skill needed to keep straight the priority of the exam preps that are necessary when scheduling a large variety of procedures each day. These tasks must be coordinated and information about them effectively communicated between the patient, the technical areas, and the physicians's office; the opportunity for error is great. This information must also be accurately entered in computerized or paper files so it is readily available for future use. Information entered by schedulers and receptionists upon interviewing the patient is often transmitted directly to the file room, where the patient's old files are retrieved for the day's work. The efficiency of the file room also depends on the schedulers: Up to two FTEs can be wasted each day chasing duplicate files or files that never existed because the initial information was not entered accurately by the schedulers. In some instances, however, this occurs because the scheduler was not able to draw out the proper information from a difficult patient.

Interpreting the physician's request or prescription is also very important, and in all instances the information on the requisition must match the physician's note. If necessary, this information should be verified with the physician's office.

Schedulers in some departments are required to perform some billing functions. Keeping track of a staggering variety of payer plans and reimbursement configurations has a significant effect not only on revenue, but also on the amount of time needed for each patient and on the skill level demanded of people collecting and deciphering this information.

In addition, schedulers and receptionists are often the first contact patients have with the department. They therefore play a key role in establishing patients' first impressions of the facility and the people who work there. Setting a positive initial impression is important because it can help develop a sense of trust and well-being in patients. This in turn puts patients in a better frame of mind as they are taken through the paces of their exams. It also improves patient cooperation, which has benefits for the technologist, and may in fact help reduce complaints about the department overall. Finally, schedulers are in frequent contact with personnel who work in referring physician's offices, and so they provide an important link to the outside world. It is not uncommon for decisions regarding where patients will be referred to be made on the basis of how this link is maintained. The reception and scheduling sections thus provide a valuable service to the department and to the patient, and their efforts are worthy of special consideration.

FILM LIBRARY SERVICES

Another radiology service that is vital to patient care is provided by file room or film library personnel. This area warehouses the hundreds of thousands to millions of films, reports, and file jackets that compose radiology medical records. The success of a film library is measured to a large degree by how often the section locates patient files and how quickly these are made available to physicians, patients, and department personnel. The file room in many ways functions as the hub of operations for the clinical sections within the department. Referring physicians often evaluate the entire department based on how well the file room functions.

As a patient arrives at the "front door" of the department for his or her study, the files should be enroute to or already at the area of the department where the exam is to be performed. Once the old films have been reviewed and the current films interpreted and reported by the radiologist, all images must be placed into the jacket and returned to the film library as soon as possible. Files will generally remain in a quick retrieval area in the main sorting area of the film library for perhaps two weeks after the study or until a few days after the patient is discharged from the hospital. Outpatient files may remain in this area for three to five days following the study. After this brief period of time, files are relocated to another area for intermediate storage.

While the reception and scheduling areas are important for making patients feel secure, the file room is usually more focused on servicing referral physicians, radiologists, and the department's clinical sections. Nothing is more upsetting to these customers than exams that are delayed or files that can't be found. This significantly affects the physician's attitude toward the hospital as well as the department.

X-ray files are medical records. As such, they are subject to specific legal requirements that must be understood and observed by file room personnel. It should be pointed out that almost all of these legal requirements are driven by state laws rather than by federal law and therefore vary from state to state. Figure 8-2 lists some of these basic legal requirements.

In addition, X-ray files must be pulled and distributed to remote areas of the hospital for countless conferences and other activities and then retrieved and refiled. Sometimes physicians or other hospital personnel do not return files from these conferences, and the file room is left to explain to an angry physician why files cannot be retrieved at the moment.

ARCHIVING FILM

Each state determines how long X-ray images must remain on file. In most states, film must remain in its original form for at least 5 years for adults or for at least 3 years after the patient reaches the age of 21. In a 400-bed community hospital that performs 120,000 exams per year, the amount of floor space needed to hold the required volume of records is approximately 7500 square feet.

Because hospital floor space is so difficult to obtain and expensive to renovate, some hospitals rent space for this purpose in low-cost storage areas that are located as far as 60 miles from the hospital. In these instances, when an archived file is needed, the warehouse receives a request via fax or phone from the department, and the files are shipped overnight to the hospital for use the next day. In other hospitals, old buildings located nearby have been renovated for film storage. In any event, the department is responsible for storing files in a safe environment. Proper environmental conditions must be considered when looking for storage space. Extremes in humidity and temperatures can damage X-ray files within a short time and render them useless; film librarians should consult with the film manufacturer for storage requirements. The hospital can be held legally accountable if proper fire protection systems are not put in place and this results in a loss of a film that affects patient treatment. Finally, the storage facility must be appropriately designed. It must have, for example, sufficient floor loading capacity. A typical stack of files five shelves high will weigh approximately 140 pounds per linear foot. This weight increases tremendously when condensed or moving stack filing systems are used. To provide reasonable assurance that structural damage will not occur, an architect or structural engineer must be consulted.

TRANSCRIPTION SERVICES

Transcription services are vital to Radiology's service program. Fast and accurate report turnaround is essential to the building and maintenance of referrals. Referring physicians must get information quickly so that they can provide treatment as soon as possible. To some degree, a patient's length of stay in the hospital is dependent on quick report turnaround time. And, if reports are late, referring physicians are put in a compromising position as their patients' queries about test results go unanswered. The JCAHO's standard is that in-

Legal Considerations for Handling Medical Records

The following items should be kept in mind when handling medical records. Medical records include X-ray reports, requisitions, and X-ray film. In fact, any documentation that routinely moves to the patient's chart or could go to the patient chart should be given careful consideration. You must keep in mind the items below are not meant to be put into practice without consultation with an appropriate individual on the facility's legal staff.

I. Who owns the medical records?

The facility owns the paper work and the X-ray images. Medical information contained in those media can be communicated to another person or facility. The facility usually has the right to retain the original records.

II. Under what circumstances can this information be communicated or released?

The information can be communicated to another person or facility only after receiving specific consent or permission from the patient or guardian to do so. This also applies when attorneys request this information.

III. How can medical information be communicated?

Teleradiography, fax, or verbal copies of images or papers can be used to send/forward this information.

VII. How long must X-rays be kept on file?

Requirements vary from state to state, but from five to seven years is typical for adults' records. For minors, images must be kept in their original form for 3 years after the patient reaches the age of 21.

Paper files such as written diagnosis, radiology requisitions, and other paper work that was once in the patient's medical file/chart must remain on hand in many states for a minimum of 10 years. For minors, these files must be available until 3 years after the patient reaches the age of 21.

V. What constitutes valid patient consent or authorization to release medical records?

It is best to have patients sign an authorization form before the files are released to the requesting party. These forms can be faxed to the patient for signature before records are released and sent back via fax to the film library. In some instances, verbal approval over the phone with a witness listening and verifying the patient's authorization is acceptable. This conversation must be documented.

It is also appropriate for the patient to show identification when choosing his or her images or records from the film library.

▶ **FIGURE 8-2** Fundamental questions regarding the handling of medical records in Radiology that have serious legal implications. (**Note:** Consult with hospital advisers before implementing medical record procedures.)

If someone other than the patient is to pick up the records, advance notice of this from the patient (and documentation) should be secured. The person picking up the records should also show identification.

VI. May patients view their own medical records?

The patient has the right to view and review his or her own medical records personally or with another individual unless the patient's physician feels this would not be in the patient's best interest. Before providing the patient with records, it is important, if not appropriate, to contact the patient's physician first and to establish the appropriateness of the patient's request.

Patients may have copies of their medical records. However, the facility has the right to assess a reasonable charge for the service. Again, it is prudent for the facility to contact the patient's physician.

VII. Subpoenas

Files requested under of a subpoena may be released without the patient's permission. A subpoena in this instance is a court order to release the records which has been signed by a judge.

▶ **FIGURE 8–2** *Continued*

patient diagnostic reports should be completed and delivered within 24 hours of the exam time. Outpatients may take longer due to reliance on the postal system. In more and more cases, however, department personnel are faxing outpatient reports directly to physicians' offices. One should keep in mind that some states have specific rules for FAXing medical records. Also, as more departments come on line with large computer systems, slave terminals are being installed in the offices of high-volume referring physicians and also on nursing floors throughout hospitals. These terminals can be used to retrieve reports that are stored electronically in the radiology department's computer system. FAX machines and printers can also be connected to the computer system and set up to receive the completed reports.

It is estimated that approximately 1200 to 1400 lines of diagnostic information will be typed each day by transcriptionists who work in a radiology department that produces 120,000 exams. An average radiology report contains about 12 to 15 lines of text. Transcriptionists' skill level must be very high in a number of distinct ways. They must learn to interpret the various dictation styles of several different radiologists. Radiologists usually dictate their findings at extremely high speed. The author has listened to tapes made by different physicians, and it is amazing how well-trained transcriptionists can interpret what sounds like rapid-fire gibberish into readable and accurate text that contains vital patient medical information. In fact, a person who already has excellent typing skills will be in training at least six months before reaching 60% of maximum productivity. In addition, the number of medical terms and variations of basic terminology that must instantaneously come to mind while listening to and transcribing dictation is extremely impressive. The most obvious skill lies in transcriptionists' typing proficiency while working with these variables.

The requirement for transcription accuracy is extremely high. One may shudder when thinking about the type of errors that can be made while transcribing reports. The omission or incorrect inclusion of a simple word such as *is* or *not* can dramatically change the meaning of a report. Today, more hospitals are considering contracting with outside companies that will receive dictation via telephone lines to their remote sites in order to improve turn-around times while keeping the service cost-effective. Such outsourcing of services are growing in popularity, and in some instances, they do offer operational and financial advantages to the department. One reason behind the superior efficiency of some outside transcription services is that they allow workers to concentrate on transcription work alone. In many radiology departments, transcriptionists also perform other tasks, such as getting reports signed, typing light correspondence, or walking to radiologists' offices to discuss questions concerning dictation. In other instances, department transcription personnel are being integrated into the hospital's medical records department to achieve improved economies of scale, while in still other situations, traditional department-based transcriptionists have been able to provide a cost-effective service and short turnaround times. Quality control efforts are usually accomplished by both the radiologist and the supervisor, who randomly selects and retains copies of typed reports and checks them against saved dictations.

COORDINATING SECTION SERVICES

Entering vital information accurately, coordinating a multitude of activities, and transmitting volumes of information properly and accurately between these nontechnical sections is key to patients' safety and to referring physicians' overall satisfaction with the radiology department's service. At a time when the availability of personnel and other resources to perform these tasks is declining, the dependency on any one employee becomes substantially greater. This is true not only in radiology, but also in every department of the hospital. Not only must speed and efficiency increase, but also accuracy cannot be compromised. This often translates into increased stress, and, if not managed appropriately, overall department efficiency will eventually decline. Departments have been losing staff in ratio to volume for the last few years due to shrinking funds because of downsizing. The department director must learn to recognize the point of diminishing returns concerning the "do more with less" philosophy and be in such position that he or she can accurately read the warning signs of excess stress and can work to maintain a reasonable productivity, and tio avoid a resource-starved environment.

CLINICAL SECTIONS AND TECHNOLOGISTS' RESPONSIBILITIES

To this point, we have described responsibilities of the nontechnical sections. As the operations of nontechnical sections suggest, we should be mindful that the range of responsibilities and the degree of skill necessary of employees goes well beyond the surface of a phone call received, a message taken, or X-ray film retrieved. It would therefore be appropriate for students to spend some time in each of these areas to gain a more detailed appreciation of the responsibility and accuracy that is required to keep these areas functioning.

Similarly, the responsibilities associated with performing a diagnostic procedure are also much greater than one might assume. The items in the list below, for example, are sometimes considered to be clerical in nature, and as a result, are sometimes ignored by technologists.

- Verify the patient's identity
- Tell the patient who you are

- Verify the significant information on the paperwork regarding the patient and the study you are to perform
- Determine the proper filming protocol
- Establish an atmosphere of professionalism
- Recognize the patient's physical condition
- Confirm with the patient what study[s] he or she is about to have and the approximate time needed
- Identify any potential for contradictions in performing the study

Reviewing these elements with each patient amounts to a brief orientation with the patient. In so many instances, the author has seen a rush to expedite the exam because of pressure to maintain high throughput. This brief introductory conversation or orientation between the patient and technologist is as a result omitted, conducted in the midst of a crowded patient area, or done in a haphazard fashion. No matter how careful reception and/or scheduling personnel may have been, information can get confused or omitted from the records, and the patient is often the best source for verifying this information. In addition, most patients expect the technologist to initiate conversation regarding these elements, and if this is not done with a degree of professionalism, the patient may feel less than confident about the amount of attention the technologist is giving the procedure. This may also reduce patient confidence in the technologist's basic skills.

In addition, helping the patient understand what to expect during the exam has been shown to reduce the probability of complaints. Informed patients are also more willing to tolerate a measure of discomfort during exams, which in turn increases their willingness to cooperate with the technologist. Also, if the technologist projects a sense of professionalism, patients are less likely to resort to seeking legal action as a result of an untoward event. However, if legal action is taken, the range of questions asked and degree of patient orientation to the procedure accomplished and documented by the technologist will help define the technologist's complicity. During the initial conversation with the patient, the technologist should let the patient know that the technologist is there to help the patient understand what is about to occur, and that questions can be asked at any time during the procedure. This gives patients a sense of confidence and a measure of security that they are not on their own.

HOW AND WHY PATIENTS COMPLAIN

In the author's experience, many patients seem to have a high threshold of physical and emotional discomfort during radiology procedures. They will hold in their feelings and express them at another time to their physicians, families, or friends. This is not necessarily due to a lack of honesty; in many cases, it is the result of fear. It is important for technologists to appreciate the mental state that is common in many patients as they arrive for their studies. Patients feel, and in fact are, very vulnerable at this time. They know that they are not in control of their circumstances, and they don't want to do anything to jeopardize the treatment or level of attention that is given by the caregiver. Sometimes, patients believe that if they make certain statements or ask certain questions, the technologist may react by not being as careful or attentive as usual during the study. In fearful situations, people are often able to contain their feelings by developing plans for escaping harm or injury or for gaining back control. It seems that the degree to which people can draw upon their experiences to accomplish one of these possibilities often helps determine how well they will handle their perceived danger. Certainly, one of these plans often includes not provoking the person who is in control. In a clinical setting, it is worthwhile for the technologist to understand that this apprehension exists at various levels in all patients during procedures. It is normal for an otherwise stable patient to become frightened and sometimes unglued by a pending diagnostic procedure. Also, in many instances, it is the fear of what tests will reveal that is of greater concern to patients. Patients often see the technologist or radiologist as someone who can influence, if not determine, the outcome of their studies, and they therefore try to be on as good terms as possible with these caregivers.

These two factors, fear of test results and perception that the caregiver may be able to affect the outcome of the test, influence how the patient will react. This is especially true when patients perceive a measure of unprofessional or improper care or conduct from the technologist, physician, or perhaps the receptionist. It is for these reasons that most often, complaints come indirectly from others after the patient leaves the hospital. Despite this indirect routing, such complaints must not be viewed as nuisances but must instead be taken seriously as opportunities to investigate objectively what actually happened and, if indicated, to find ways to make improvements. In the author's experience, working openly with department supervisors to make improvements based on these complaints can actually strengthen team spirit within the department, especially when recognition is given when the problem is corrected.

LOOKING FOR TROUBLE CAN HELP THE PATIENT

It is extremely easy for the technologist to lose sight of the patient when working in a maze of wheelchairs, stretchers, cassettes, paperwork, and X-ray machines. This is particularly true in the midst of general activity in a busy diagnostic area. However, it is necessary for the technologist to be alert and to be aware that important bits of information may not be present and need clarification. During the brief patient orientation discussed above, the patient may have indicated a detail inconsistent with the exam that is to be performed. Perhaps some signal draws the warning that the study that has been ordered may be at variance with the patient's condition, drug sensitivity, past illness, or disability which was not recorded. This may affect the appropriateness or timeliness of the exam at hand and could even have an impact on the patient's well-being. The author can recall more than one instance that if it were not for the technologist's keen attention to some of these details, a patient's well-being would have been compromised.

THE TECHNOLOGIST AS MARKETING AGENT

The technologist plays another important role in the overall success and effectiveness of the radiology service. As we discussed in earlier chapters, signing contracts with payers is an extremely important factor in maintaining patient volume. Providing accurate diagnoses is not necessarily the primary reason payers will write contracts with hospitals or private offices; the service element is also seriously considered. Figure 8-3 outlines factors that influence the service element of a radiology department. Technologists must realize the importance of their role and their individual efforts.

The author has observed many times technologists losing sight of the fact that the patient must be the focus of our attention. The simple logistics of transporting or escorting the patient from point to point in the department can distract our observation of basic patient needs. In fact, sometimes it appears that we perceive the patient to be an obstacle to the fulfillment of our primary mission of meeting productivity standards rather than focus on the level of service we are actually there to provide. It takes little extra time and effort to keep

---

Fundamental Elements of Service

I. Convenience: The ease with which customers can make use of the services provided. The "user-friendly" character of policies, procedures, hours of operations, and limitations that are characteristic of the facility.

II. Friendliness: The manner in which customers are approached, helped, and led through directions and the procedures to be completed.

III. Cost of service: Cost of service must be viewed as being in balance with services provided elsewhere given the degree to which the elements of service overall are carried out.

IV. Quality: There should be a high degree of reliability and accuracy of the medical information and outcome patients receive from services.

V. Follow-up: There should be a mechanism through which contact with the patient is made in a fashion that is appropriate to the intensity or nature of service provided. This could range from direct phone contact with patients after the service was rendered to random mailings of satisfaction survey forms.

▶ **FIGURE 8–3** Shows factors that influence the service element of a radiology department.

the patient's needs clearly in focus while dealing with these distractions. Benefits to the technologist lie in increased patient confidence in the technologist's skills, which makes the patient more cooperative. This also increases the technologist's self-confidence and adds value to the department and hospital.

VALUE-ADDED EFFORT BY DEPARTMENT EMPLOYEES

From a general management perspective, technologists who develop positive work habits when working with patients and can keep their focus on details and on maintaining a positive service orientation are more valuable to the department. This assumes, of course, that the individual has also achieved an acceptable level of technical competence. In short, superior technical competence or expertise will not compensate for a lack of patient-focused skills. In the health care profession, people skills, adaptability, compassion, and accuracy are primary requirements if career advancement is of interest. Developing people skills to be used with peers and radiologists as well as patient management skills is vital for career advancement, and those who pay attention to these factors will become recognized employees.

PUTTING IT TOGETHER: THE ORGANIZATION'S CULTURE

Each department in an organization develops a culture or personality that is the sum of the values and philosophies held by the people in that department. This personality or culture can be readily detected by anyone who enters the department. An example of this is how comfortable we feel being in a store based on the perceived character of the sales clerks and on the store's appearance and layout. Patients can sense an organization's culture, and perhaps the level of quality that will be provided. Another indicator is the manner in which the employees handle both routine and unusual situations that involves a patient.

Culture is not necessarily driven by an organization's size, the volume of services it provides, or by how sophisticated its equipment is. It is driven by the philosophies and value system recognized by those who work there. In many instances, the seeds that grow into and encourage the value system, philosophies, and many other aspects of the department are both sown and limited by management. Department culture will certainly have a bearing on the quality of care that is provided and on the style with which it is delivered. In most cases patients can feel this culture and will react accordingly. Patients will in general react more positively to any given circumstance in an environment where the culture supports a positive and friendly orientation. It is the management's responsibility to provide direction toward such a culture and the responsibility of the department employees to recognize its potential value.

Other considerations regarding department culture are not patient- or service-oriented. As a technologist in training, you may have relatively few choices when selecting a clinical site for employment. However, understanding the culture of a department when seeking employment is an important part of looking for employment. Joining a positive organizational culture that allows employees to feel good about their participation in and contribution to the total effort can have an important impact on your career.

Establishing a positive culture clearly begins with the leadership of an organization, but maintaining a positive and helpful environment also places some responsibility on its employees. One characteristic of a positive work environment is that employees understand the goals and values of the organization and can relate what they do to those goals and values.

ESTABLISHING GOALS AND PERFORMANCE STANDARDS

Operational goals and standards are worthy of serious consideration. Clearly, these operational goals should apply to all health care facilities regardless of size or setting:

- Increased efficiency of personnel
- Minimized patient delays
- Reduced incidence of and potential for patient injury
- Reduced incidence of and potential for patient inconvenience
- Improved level of professionalism of the service
- More positive and livable work environment for department employees

Patients have a right to expect a high degree of attention to these goals. As noted earlier, one recognizable department goal should be that department personnel view the patient as the object of their principal interest and not as an obstacle to achieving procedural, quality, productivity, or technical goals. This is certainly not an easy task; however, it can be achieved if sections are well coordinated and if section goals are defined and prioritized in a fashion that everyone can understand.

OPERATIONAL PLANS, "ORG" CHARTS, AND POLICIES

A significant part of an operating plan is the department's organization chart. For large departments that have sections with more than one layer of supervision, an organization chart for the section may be helpful. The department's organization chart defines the various sections and clarifies their relationships within the organization. Organization charts are helpful because they help clarify reporting lines and help define supervisors' span of control.

REVIEWING POLICIES PERIODICALLY TO ENSURE COORDINATED SERVICES

The ongoing level of activity in a section along with the repetition of daily routine can over time give rise to a false sense of how well employees actually understand operational policies and procedures in a section. Diversity of policy interpretation by employees usually becomes apparent when specific procedures are discussed in detail at group meetings. Often, procedures are "modified" by each employee as time passes. This is sometimes because employees believe that such small adjustments to or changes in procedure are actually more effective than the details of a written procedure. As a result, employees begin to work out of synch with each other and errors and/or subtle inefficiencies begin to creep into the service. This will impact section performance and increase the probability of errors and inefficiencies. A periodic review and, if indicated, updating of long-standing policies that govern even the most basic procedures can be helpful. If policies are revised, it is important to verify their compatibility with the current operations of other sections in the department and, in some instances, with other departments in the hospital. New or revised policies must be appropriately developed through discussions with staff, supervisors, radiologists, and the department director.

Section objectives should be realistically calibrated to match the level of resources available. Section objectives should also support the department's mission statement and overall department goals. In turn, each manager should understand the department's mission statement, which is often written by the department director in conjunction with the chairperson and, in some instances, the hospital VP. If operations in another section obstruct a section from meeting its realistic goals, the supervisor and department director must develop strategies and work with these sections to provide necessary compatibility and support.

The section's objectives and mission statement can then be used as a baseline against which current and future services and activities can be gauged. The quality of the section's objectives and mission statement will in part indicate the value system and the culture of the organization and the probability that that organization will achieve its goals. The sum of these factors becomes the section's, and, ultimately, the department's service plan.

Simply having these administrative and operations tools in place will not assure the success of a given service or of the organization as a whole. A service plan provides a blueprint for success, may help generate the involvement of employees, and encourages a more positive attitude about executing the plan by clarifying long-standing uncertainties about specific responsibilities of personnel and procedures. But each employee must be encouraged to take an equal share in this effort and must accept specific responsibilities contributing to its success.

THE FUNDAMENTAL FORMAT OF A DEPARTMENT ORGANIZATION CHART

As we saw in Chapter Seven, an organization chart is a pictorial representation of an organization's management structure. Organization charts can show a flat or a vertical management structure. A flat management structure has few midlevel supervisory or management positions. In today's economy, flat structures are becoming necessary because they represent a more efficient operation with fewer management people and lower administrative costs. The operational implication is that it forces responsibility for decision making to fewer people. Even more importantly, it forces decisions to be made at a point closer to where the work is being done, that is, among first-line supervisors and employees. A flat organization structure tends to increase effectiveness in decision making because fewer decision makers are involved. The immediate effect is that there is a higher dependency on each manager or supervisor to make decisions and to cooperate effectively with employees regarding the outcome. The flat format also stimulates growth and vigor among management people, who become empowered to make decisions and to perform at a higher level. Also, with fewer managers, communication lines becomes more direct and less cumbersome. There is no question that this format can have a beneficial effect on the services the department offers its patients and medical staff.

THE LINK BETWEEN RADIOLOGY AND OTHER HOSPITAL SERVICES

As noted earlier, there are very few if any radiology departments that still operate as separate concessions. Departments today operate as extensions of hospital administration, not as separate entities. The extension of the hospital administration reaches into the department through various department managers and supervisors. The department director usually reports to the hospital through the vice president of clinical services. The VP responsible for Radiology also manages other departments, and his or her authority includes obtaining operational and budgetary approval for these departments.

HOSPITAL–DEPARTMENT POLITICS

In addition to attending to the department's operational responsibilities, it is equally important for the department director to maintain a positive working relationship with other department directors in the hospital as well as with all levels of the hospital administration. These latter relationships can be significantly affected by the department's culture and by the effectiveness of service the department provides.

Relationships with other departments also have important operational implications (Fig. 8-4). It is imperative that all departments within the hospital function together with a high degree of coordination and cooperation. It is also imperative that when coordination between departments begins to weaken or fail, the appropriate directors work together effectively to reach effective solutions. Diplomacy and skill are needed to work through problems that involve more than one department. The success of such discussions will impact the hospital's overall efficiency and cost-effectiveness. The expectations and efforts of each participant must be discussed and positive results attained.

MANAGEMENT MEETINGS, OBJECTIVES, AND MISSION STATEMENTS

By now, you can see that putting it all together so a given department can provide the best overall service possible is dependent on many elements, including operational processes, management expertise, individual effort of its employees, and financial resources. The effort is also held together by regularly scheduled department management meetings. One method of assuring communication among sections is to hold operations or management meetings regularly with department supervisors. Such meetings may be scheduled weekly,

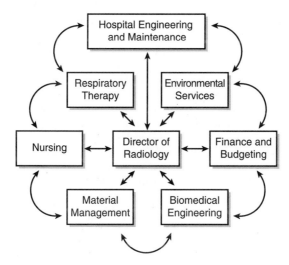

▶ **FIGURE 8-4** Shows the various channels of communication among department directors that are necessary. These communication patterns must be developed and maintained over long periods of time. Keeping effective communication continuing in a productive fashion requires a great deal of diplomacy and creativity so that operations problems can be anticipated and corrected before department stereotyping and an unhealthy degree of territorial competition occurs.

biweekly, or monthly depending on the complexity and needs of the department. The frequency of these meetings is affected by the sheer volume of activity or number of issues that need to be discussed on an ongoing basis. It is important that these meetings function in a cordial but businesslike manner and that an agenda is used and minutes are taken and then distributed. Attendees should include the department director and an appropriate mix of supervisors and managers. Such an operations group may have as few as 2 or as many as 12 members.

Operational meetings create a forum to discuss formally a wide variety of management and budget issues. They can also provide a positive reinforcement tool that can help managers and supervisors understand and keep tuned in to the department's central set of goals and standards of performance. In the author's experience, these meetings can be enhanced by designating some time for educational programs which may be presented by non-Radiology personnel, for instance people in key hospital departments such as finance, human resources, and the legal department. Information sessions such as these not only help keep department managers informed, but also send an important signal to the rest of the hospital that the Radiology management group is keeping up with new information and is not operating in a vacuum. In addition, hospital administrators and other presenters have an opportunity to establish their identities and credibility with the department's supervisors. Such meetings also put the department's management group in a position to demonstrate their professionalism, to ask questions and get worthwhile information about what is happening outside the department, and to engage in beneficial discussions that otherwise might not have occurred.

As the director's efforts to coordinate services with other hospital departments continue, each section in Radiology must learn to operate both as a unique entity and as an entity inextricably bound to other sections both inside and outside of Radiology. A sense of territorial rights as well as prejudices among section supervisors should be encouraged to a reasonable degree to build each section's identity as a team. However, these must be tempered when they begin to distract from the overall radiology program.

On a practical level, it is how difficulties between sections are eventually handled by department management and individual employees that provides some indication of the department's success. Intramural operational difficulties can be handled either as an opportunity to improve operations or as a signal to employees that they should circle the wagons and protect their own immediate interests. In the former exists an opportunity for growth and improvement, and in the latter exists an opportunity for entrenchment and continued defensive posturing, which creates disharmony and a loss of service.

STUDY QUESTIONS

1. Select four separate sections of Radiology and provide the following information for each section.

   Fundamental function

   Opportunities for errors by employees and how these affect patient care. Give a hypothetical circumstance to clarify your answer.

   Specific functions that can generate stress for the employee

2. By using at least two examples, explain why it is important for each section to function as a separate unit but also to operate in synchronization with all other department sections.

3. List the elements a technologist should cover with a patient before an exam gets under way. Briefly comment on why each of these elements is important to cover.

4. While in the exam room with the patient, and even during the procedure, what should the technologist do to keep the patient informed and to what degree should general conversation with the patient go on?

5. Do you think it is appropriate for an employee to accept the role of marketing agent as he or she fulfills his or her routine responsibilities? Briefly explain your views.

6. Briefly explain how you can use some aspects of your personality to improve communication with the patient before, during, and after the study. Consider that you will be dealing with patients in more than one age group and who have different abilities to cooperate and respond to your actions.

7. Briefly describe your understanding of the organizational pecking order and how a department's standing is established. What can a department do to improve this standing?

8. List the various elements you would want to address when writing a section operating plan, and briefly explain why you would want to include them in your plan.

9. Briefly describe what you understand about organizational culture, how it affects service to the patient, and its implications with regard to your selection of future employers.

Radiology Management

OBJECTIVES FOR STUDY

After reading this chapter, the student will

▶ Understand the basic steps involved in developing a department budget.

▶ Understand the fundamental terminology needed to work with budgets.

▶ Understand the basic information needed to develop a capital budget.

▶ Appreciate the basic steps involved in developing equipment purchase proposal requests and bid criteria.

▶ Appreciate the concepts basic to personnel management and motivation.

▶ Appreciate the concepts basic to developing a salary scale.

▶ Appreciate various management styles.

INTRODUCTION

In Chapters Seven and Eight, we covered several operational topics that are very much a part of providing a high-quality and efficient radiology service. In this chapter, we will look at a few other aspects of radiology management in more detail. Questions regarding budget development and general management will be explored to provide a more complete view of Radiology operations. We will also touch upon some of the management theories associated with motivation and management style, which may help the reader understand the basics of successful processes and operational programs. We will begin by discussing one of the most important aspects of Radiology management: finalizing the budget.

PREPARING THE OPERATING AND CAPITAL BUDGETS

Table 9-1 shows a budget variance report for a radiology department. As we discussed in Chapter Four, budgets are composed of line items which help sort out specific expenditures. Many discrete purchases from several different suppliers may be included in one line item. The finance department at each hospital defines the titles of line items slightly differently, but, in general, they follow a fairly predictable pattern. Actual titles and methods for categorizing various income and expense activities within line items don't matter so long as they are understood by department personnel, the purchasing department, and the finance department. Such understanding is essential; otherwise purchases and other expenses will not be tagged with the correct account (line item) number and tracked on future budget report sheets. There may be times when a single purchase or expense is in itself unique or so significant that the finance department will approve its own line number. Examples are X-ray film and some service contracts.

Expense line items are typically expenses that are internally charged by one department of the hospital to another. For instance, clinical engineering may charge Radiology for repair work performed or the maintenance department may charge Radiology for the installation of cabinets. In some hospitals, Radiology's portion of facility overhead expenses for heat, electricity, water, and the general depreciation of floor space the department occupies may be charged, although this is not a common practice. In many hospitals, overhead expenses do appear in the plant manager's budget.

Preparing the Budget

The first formal step toward preparing the department budget is to schedule budget meetings with each section of the department. The purpose of a budget meeting is to review in detail the items below:

1. Volume of activity
2. Changes in prices of supplies
3. Changes in scope of services
4. Changes in personnel expenses
5. Changes in equipment needed

After much review and some follow-up discussions with supervisors, radiologists, and the chairperson, the department director should have all the potential operational issues in mind and will be able to understand how they will affect the upcoming year's expenses. This information will then be translated into discrete monetary values and allocat-

EXPENSE/REVENUE BUDGET COMPARISON (WHOLE DOLLAR)

EXPENSE	CURRENT MONTH				YEAR TO DATE			
	Actual	Budget	Variance	% Variance	Actual	Budget	Variance	% Variance
001 Salaries	142,955	135,377	7,578	5.6	1,192,602	1,120,706	71,896	6.4
003 Salaries-Nursing Rm	1,151	0	1,151	.0	10,417	0	10,417	.0
027 Physician Fees	0	0	0	.0	0	0	0	.0
390 Medical Supplies	50,854	35,815	15,039	42.0	381,735	322,334	59,401	18.4
395 Film and Processing	87,741–	29,167	116,908–	400.8–	177,344	262,499	85,155–	32.4–
460 Office Supplies	4,573	3,638	935	25.7	30,704	32,742	2,038–	6.2–
490 Minor Equipment	2,370	709	1,661	234.3	11,596	6,373	5,223	82.0
500 Uniforms and Scrubs	0	0	0	.0	0	0	0	.0
560 Service Contracts	12,800	19,562	6,762–	34.6–	149,282	176,058	26,776–	15.2–
570 Repairs and Maintenance	58,915	7,500	51,415	685.5	228,333	67,500	160,833	238.3
600 Purchased service	12,533	5,200	7,333	141.0	398,920	301,200	97,720	32.4
650 Advertising	586	600	14–	2.3–	1,400	5,400	4,000–	74.1–
770 Leases and Rentals	79,066	32,267	46,799	145.0	317,063	290,399	26,664	9.2
890 Dues and Subscriptions	700	359	341	95.0	3,278	3,223	55	1.7
920 Travel and Education	205	0	205	.0	5,665	0	5,665	.0
930 Misc Supplies and Expenses	233	1,200	967–	80.6–	3,451	10,800	7,349–	68.0–
950 Freight	776	1,000	224–	22.4–	2,842	9,000	6,158–	68.4–
Total	279,976	272,394	7,582	2.8	2,914,634	2,608,234	306,400	11.7

Shows a variance report for a radiology department.

ed to budget line items. To make these line item estimates, the following steps should be taken:

1. Review last year's budget and actual expenses and understand the year-end variances

2. Understand the volume of work performed and how that volume related to actual expenses (i.e., cost per exam)

3. Anticipate volume for the coming year

4. Anticipate any changes (expansion, addition, or deletion) in programs

5. Review the above with the supervisor and radiologists in detail to give everyone an opportunity to understand the previous year's costs and the assumptions for the coming year

6. Calculate new volume projections against the current ratio of expenses for each line item

7. Calculate in special inflation factors over those already incurred by the hospital as needed

It is extremely important to gather all information that may be related to the items outlined above before filling in the blanks on the budget work sheet. The information-gathering phase, or prep work, is very time consuming and more demanding than it may appear to the causal observer. Notes should be taken at the budget meeting to document what has been said and what commitments have been made by those around the table. Commitments to increased volume or decreased expenses should be noted and used as benchmarks for measuring the performance of managers, supervisors, and radiologists. In fact, all the activities involved in preparing the budget should be ongoing throughout the year, and follow-up discussions should be scheduled when actual budget performance is not meeting commitments.

Variable and Fixed Operating Expenses

It is helpful to understand a few basic terms as we look through the various budget sheets presented in this chapter. The first of these is *variable expenses*. These are operating expenses that fluctuate with volume, and they must be budgeted accordingly. Examples of variable expenses are X-ray film and film-processing chemistry. When estimating variable expenses for the year, calculations are made on the basis of unit cost multiplied by volume. Obviously, more patient volume will require more film. Generally these calculations can be done by working with percentages. If overall volume is expected to go up in CT, for example, by 10%, one can usually safely project that film costs will increase by 10% also. There are some secondary issues that must be understood, however, before one can feel comfortable with predicting a cost increase of 10%:

1. Are any changes in filming protocols anticipated that will change the number of films needed per case?

2. Are any changes in basic film costs that are charged by the supplier anticipated?

3. Is there likely to be a change in the number of extra copies of images sent to referring physicians, the ED, or ICU floors for their use and convenience?

If the answer to any of these questions is yes, the expenses associated with this variable must be detailed and calculated into the 10% volume assumption.

Costs that are not directly associated with volume are known as *fixed costs*. An example of a fixed cost item is expenses for equipment service contracts. In general, the price of a service contract will remain the same throughout the year whether a piece of equipment performs 5000 or 7000 exams in a given year. For the most part, personnel costs are considered to be fixed costs even though some elements, such as overtime, will vary somewhat depending on volume or other circumstances. More recently, staffing plans are being built around fluctuating demand. If this becomes standard practice, one may consider staffing a variable expense more seriously.

We discussed depreciation expenses in Chapter Four. Depreciation expenses are generally calculated by the finance department on buildings and equipment throughout the hospital and will usually not appear on department work sheets.

Each expense for each line item must be reviewed taking into account the basic questions and circumstances noted earlier. It is imperative to have a good understanding of how referring physicians' practicing patterns may change during the upcoming year. For example, a group of cardiologists may anticipate for various reasons a significant change in the number of nuclear medicine stress referrals. This anticipation may be based on the fact that the practice has just been awarded or just lost a large provider contract. This change in volume will affect personnel and supply expenses for the nuclear medicine section. Or, for instance, a practice may anticipate taking on a physician who has experience and expertise in evaluating bone density in women. This could affect either the CT schedule or the need for a new bone density scanner. Such information can be gathered reasonably well by department radiologists, who usually have conversations throughout the year with a wide range of medical staff about their individual practice plans. Also, supervisors in the department will often hear about such changes directly or indirectly from various members of the medical staff. In short, information such as this can be very important to the department's success rate in anticipating volume and variations in operating expenses for the coming year. In fact, the amount of time spent on this sort of investigation and prep work, rather than the actual calculation of numbers, actually accounts for most of the effort involved in preparing the budget.

Direct and *indirect expenses* are other commonly used terms. Direct expenses include costs that are directly associated with the principal activity of a cost center. For example, let us define the ultrasound section as a cost center (an operation that has its own budget or account), and we will identify this cost center as account number 725. All expenses associated with ultrasound activity will be shown under this account number. An example of a direct expense for this account or cost center is film, because film expenses are directly associated with the principal activity of the section. Personnel is another example a direct expense. In most cases, direct expenses can also be variable expenses.

Indirect expenses have a slightly different character, but they are still vital to the service. Examples of indirect expenses are telephone expenses, service contracts, and cleaning services. Indirect expenses can be variable or fixed expenses.

The Capital Budget and Acquisition of Major Equipment

Acquisition of major equipment is vital to the long-term efficiency and success of radiology departments. Equipment acquisition can be divided into four distinct steps (1) budgeting, (2) developing bid specifications, (3) negotiating the terms of purchase, and (4) installation and formal acceptance. Figure 9-1 shows a flowchart for capital equipment acquisition.

Budgeting Capital Expenses

There are three basic reasons for acquiring capital equipment. The first is to replace equipment, the second is to acquire additional equipment, and the third is to acquire new

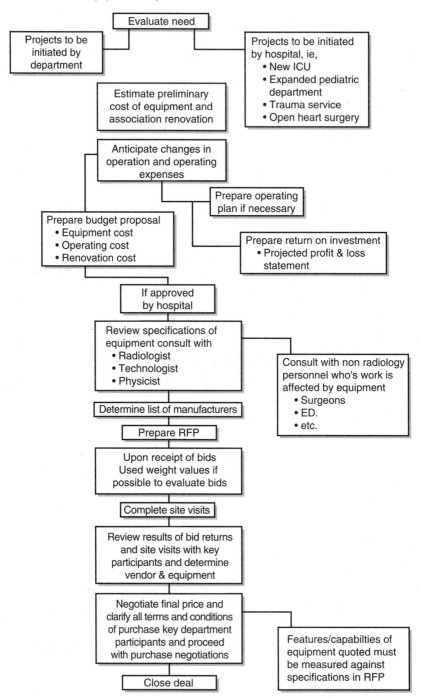

Equipment Acquisition Process

Evaluate need

Projects to be initiated by department

Projects to be initiated by hospital, ie,
- New ICU
- Expanded pediatric department
- Trauma service
- Open heart surgery

Estimate preliminary cost of equipment and association renovation

Anticipate changes in operation and operating expenses

Prepare operating plan if necessary

Prepare budget proposal
- Equipment cost
- Operating cost
- Renovation cost

Prepare return on investment
- Projected profit & loss statement

If approved by hospital

Review specifications of equipment consult with
- Radiologist
- Technologist
- Physicist

Consult with non radiology personnel who's work is affected by equipment
- Surgeons
- ED.
- etc.

Determine list of manufacturers

Prepare RFP

Upon receipt of bids Used weight values if possible to evaluate bids

Complete site visits

Review results of bid returns and site visits with key participants and determine vendor & equipment

Negotiate final price and clarify all terms and conditions of purchase key department participants and proceed with purchase negotiations

Features/capabilties of equipment quoted must be measured against specifications in RFP

Close deal

▶ **FIGURE 9–1** The equipment acquisition process includes many aspects that are often overlooked, especially given the effort to reduce capital costs and their associated operating costs. Background information from several sources both outside and inside Radiology must be captured and carefully factored into capital requests.

▶ TABLE 9–2
CAPITAL-BUDGET REQUEST SUMMARY

Department: Radiology   1994

ITEM DESCRIPTION	FAC (F) OR EQUIP (E)	QUANTITY	NEW (N) or REPLACE (R)	TOTAL COST
GI R/F X-ray Machine	E	1	R	$475,000
GI Network Software	E	1	N	$25,000
MRI 5 X Upgrade	E	2	Upgrade	715,000
MRI Phased Array Hardware	E	2	Upgrade	240,000
Magnetic Tape Drives	E	5	R	15,000
Coil Modification Kit	E	1	N	$5,000
Neuro CT, Network Connection CT Scanner	E	1	N	$15,500
NM Laser Imager W' Network Connections	E	1	R	$115,000
NM Triple Head Scanner	E	1	R	$475,000
Ulsd Patient Exam Tables	E	8	R	$40,000
Angio Addl' Disk Storage	E	1	Upgrade	$50,000
Bone/Chest Portable C-Arm	E	1	R	$115,000
CT Scanner				$1,200,000
RIS Disk Storage, and Barcode Readers	E	Mtpl Units	R	$100,000
Relocation & Comp Connections/Bus Off	F			$50,000
Diagnostic Service Equipment	E	3	R/N	$10,000
Patient Monitoring & Resuscitation Equip	E	6	R/N	$45,000
Page Total				$3,690,500

Medical Director _____   Chairman _____
Assoc Administrator _____

Shows a typical summary of radiology capital budget requests.

technology. Each hospital applies its own philosophy and criteria to the approval of these purchases, but because of the changing economic environment, the hospital's criteria for approving equipment purchases may change slightly each year. Capital expenses also include any renovation and building expenses, which may or may not be associated with equipment purchases. Depending on the criteria and format required by the hospital, capital budget packages can be among the most voluminous documents generated by a department. They may contain 15 to 20 pages of forms, text, and related background information, and as Table 9-2 shows, department requests for capital expenditures can total in the millions of dollars. Capital expenses for Radiology make up a significant portion of most hospitals' overall capital budgets. A hospital's annual capital budget's expenses might range from $6 to $12 million. Depending on the hospital's mission and other current circumstances, the radiology department at a 400-bed community hospital, for example, might require $2.5 to $3.5 million in equipment and renovation expenses and be approved for $1.5 or $2.5 million in expenditures. With such a significant share of the capital expense pie going to Radiology, plenty of support documentation reflecting department management care and prudence is usually included in the annual package of capital requests.

Budgeting for Replacement Equipment

As we mentioned earlier, approval to replace equipment is generally straightforward. However, issues that may still need to be addressed satisfactorily are:

1. Present age of equipment compared to life expectancy
2. Utilization (this can be expressed as time of actual use as a percentage of a nine-hour work day
3. Downtime and actual service cost and work history
4. Availability of replacement parts
5. Safety of equipment (electrical, mechanical, and radiation)
6. Obsolescence based on capabilities to perform current and foreseeable future exams
7. One-of-a-kind status

These criteria have no special priority. Depending on circumstances, answers to the questions associated with only one or two of the seven may indicate a worthwhile reason to warrant equipment replacement. In the past, most requests for replacement equipment met little challenge; however, in today's economic environment, these requests are much more seriously evaluated.

Budgeting for Additional Equipment

The department director must anticipate a great deal of scrutiny from hospital administrators before they approve requests for additional capital equipment. In some instances, requests for duplicate equipment must address a slightly different set of issues than those for other equipment:

1. Utilization of existing equipment that is available to perform like-kind exams
2. Location of like-kind equipment in the department/building
3. What change in demand for service has occurred
4. What is the anticipated utilization of this equipment over the first 6, 12, and 18 months
5. Percentage of in- and outpatient exams that will be performed with the new machine
6. How will this new equipment affect the operating budget?

Here again, there is no particular hierarchy of criteria that, if satisfied, will automatically result in approval. Answers to questions associated with these issues must lead to a logical determination that service and/or efficiency requirements will be appropriately satisfied.

We should also keep in mind that requesting fewer items than needed can actually cause more problems than can overbudgeting. Hospital decisions to add new services may not appear at first to affect capital expenses in Radiology. But, for example, additional critical care beds can leave radiology technologists frustrated all year as requesting physicians complain about slow response time resulting from not having enough portable equipment immediately ready for use. An expansion of the OR may require consideration of additional C-Arm equipment. A new physician brought on staff by the hospital to develop and expand services involving diagnosis of endocrine system disorders may require additional CT or MR services. This new service alone would not require an additional scanner. However, if the associated radiology services are already stretched to the limit, additional referrals may require at least an addition 3-D image reconstruction work station in Radiology or perhaps the addition of special MRI coils. Such a work station will cost approximately $250,000, and MRI coils often cost from $10,000 to $20,000. If such additions are not planned for, the hospital may have to take funds from its contingency budget. It is incumbent upon the radiology department director to keep as informed as possible about new hospital programs so that appropriate imaging services support will be available when needed. This information can be obtained through casual conversations with radiologists, directors of various departments throughout the hospital, and members of the hospital medical staff. Hospital news bulletins are another source of such information.

Budgeting for New Technology

The third type of capital request may involve implementation of a new service and purchase of new technology. Let's use breast biopsy–localization equipment and angioplasty equipment as examples of this. New programs almost always involve:

1. Changes in personnel
2. Renovations
3. Purchases of both large and small capital equipment items
4. A new or revised operating budget

In order to understand the details of and to justify a new program, a business plan is needed. A business plan is a comprehensive explanation of all aspects of the proposed program. It contains information about cost, purpose, and other integral elements, as described in Figure 9-2. These elements are usually defined after a careful review of the financial, personnel, operations, and any political issues that may arise from its introduction and implementation. Such a program may involve the integration of two radiology services or the separation of two services that had been integrated. It may involve a new technology or a new freestanding outpatient facility. In any case, a considerable degree of new research and planning is needed, and the business plan documents and addresses all these issues.

The business plan is usually presented as part of the department's capital budget package. The project itself may receive funding through the usual department capital request process, or it may be funded by other sources. Certainly, requesting new radiology programs in today's environment must be done with special care if they are to have any chance for approval.

Budgeting for Plant Expenditures

A fourth type of capital request involves improvements or changes to the physical plant. Justification here is relatively straightforward, and the following issues must be addressed to establish need:

1. Improve efficiency of personnel
2. Improve aesthetics of area
3. Improve privacy or comfort of patients
4. Meet building code requirements
5. Improve safety of area

It is always important to provide as much worthwhile background information as possible. Table 9-3 shows a typical equipment inventory schedule, which helps orient administration and board members to the type of equipment that is available. Other schedules can

**Business Plan
Financial Analysis
and
Facility and Operations Assessment
Shady Side Freestanding Radiology Facility**

I. Introduction

Provide a brief summary of reason for this service and a sense of the size and complexity of the project.

II. Personnel Assessment

Describe overall scope of service and summarize need for projected staff. Discuss special considerations that may exist regarding scheduling.

III. Equipment Assessment

Describe the nature of equipment that will be needed to handle the anticipated volume.
Discuss special considerations regarding equipment needs.

IV. Operating Hours

Discuss demand for the service. Cover the relative need to operate during evening or weekend hours.

V. Image Interpretation and Transcription

Develop turnaround time standards and describe the routing of reports.

VI. Summary of Miscellaneous Start-Up Costs

Summarize all unusual start-up costs that are shown in the financial tables listed below.

VII. Financial Tables

Table I   Projected Volume Assessment
Table IIA   Payer Mix and Collection Rate
Table IIB   Payer Mix and Collection Rate
Table III   Current Outpatient Volume and Exam Mix
Table IV   Projected Equipment Costs
Table V   Projected Minor Equipment Needs
Table VI   Return on Investment Calculations

VIII. Assessment of Other Reasonable Alternatives

Discuss all reasonable alternatives to implementing the proposed plan. Carefully describe how and when other plans could be implemented, and why these plans have not been recommended.

▶ **FIGURE 9-2** Table of contents for a typical business plan.

▶ TABLE 9-3
CAPITAL EQUIPMENT INVENTORY

DESCRIPTION AND NOTATIONS	COST	CONSTRUCTION COSTS	COMBINED COSTS	YEAR INSTALLED	PRESENT AGE	YEAR POST DEPRECIATION	SCHEDULED YEAR TO REPLACE	LIFE
Gen Rad #1	$170,000	$5,000	$175,000	1974	20	−12	1982	8
Angio #1	$700,000	$50,000	$750,000	1986	8	−2	1992	6
RIS Comp Sys	$500,000	$5,000	$505,000	1971	23	−15	1979	8
R/F Unit #4	$650,000	$100,000	$750,000	1985	9	−2	1992	7
CT Body #1	$1,300,000	$75,000	$1,375,000	1988	6	0	1994	6
Scanner, N.M. #2	$450,000	$5,000	$455,000	1985	9	−3	1991	6
Portable #1	$42,000	$0	$42,000	1984	10	−4	1990	6
Portable #2	$42,000	$0	$42,000	1986	8	−2	1992	6
Portable #3	$42,000	$0	$42,000	1979	15	−9	1985	6
Mammo Ulsd	$90,000	$5,000	$95,000	1987	7	−1	1993	6
Skull & General #4	$265,000	$50,000	$315,000	1976	18	−10	1984	8
Gen #2	$350,000	$25,000	$375,000	1976	18	−11	1983	7
Mammo	$90,000	$5,000	$95,000	1986	8	0	1994	8
Ulsd #1	$350,000	$5,000	$355,000	1986	8	−2	1992	6
Ulsd #2	$350,000	$2,000	$352,000	1985	9	−3	1991	6
Ulsd #3	$350,000	$2,000	$352,000	1987	7	−1	1993	6
Total	$6,571,000	$344,000	$6,915,000					

An inventory of major capital equipment.

229

be used to help them understand why capital requests are being made. Equipment being used beyond its life expectancy is usually not in and of itself an appropriate reason to replace equipment. However, an equipment depreciation schedule can help to establish the average age of major equipment in the department and show that implementing a prudent equipment replacement program would be wiser than waiting for these items to cause service problems. Such a schedule would also indicate how to estimate service contract expenses on the older units as well as help to predict total future service costs and downtime problems. In addition, it is very advisable to have a comprehensive and detailed accounting of service records so that a strong case can be made when the time is right to replace a particular machine.

Many elements enter into the process of budgeting for capital equipment. There are a few important steps that must be completed before a department budget can be put together with reasonable expectations for success, and several of these were already covered when we discussed pre-budget discussions for the operating budget. We must keep in mind that although the operating budget and the capital budget are very different in nature, they are in some ways interdependent. Because of this, it is important that capital and operating budget issues be discussed thoroughly at one budget meeting as described earlier in the chapter. The important points to be made here are that it is the department director's responsibility to keep his or her antennae up throughout the year to minimize the element of surprise and that budgeting is not a process that occurs during only the last three months of the fiscal year.

Before any requests are even listed on paper, focused discussions must be conducted throughout the department. Discussion with clerical people, radiologists, and technologists about equipment or renovation needs should occur. During these meetings, a careful review of activity during the previous year should take place. In addition, discussions regarding new hospital programs that may be under review should be covered. Also, current equipment needs within the section should be considered, and, finally, how all of these issues may be affected by other services the hospital is considering must be evaluated.

Approval of Nonbudgeted Capital Equipment

There are times when an equipment purchase is necessary but has not been budgeted. To cover these situations, hospitals generally maintain a capital contingency fund. The amount of money in this fund is allocated by the board and varies with hospital size. A 400-bed hospital may have a contingency fund of $300,000 to $400,000. At times, the board may approve a relatively high allocation if special circumstances are foreseen for the coming year. When nonbudgeted capital equipment is needed, a formal request must be submitted with appropriate documentation. In general, using contingency money, particularly early in the fiscal year, is not viewed favorably. There are circumstances in which unbudgeted purchases could not have been anticipated. In other instances, an item that has been provisionally approved by the regular capital budget program may be purchased if certain prerequisite circumstances in fact occur later in the fiscal year. Requests for contingency capital funds are generally reviewed first by hospital administration for need and appropriateness and then presented to the board for review and final approval.

Shopping for Capital Equipment and Preparing the Request for Proposal (RFP)

After a capital item has been approved, the department must make plans to evaluate which equipment manufacturer has equipment that will best meet the department's needs. There are many approaches to this step, but they should all include the following elements:

1. A discussion with the ordering physician to verify future service needs
2. A discussion with radiologists to identify service equipment operational requirements, capabilities, and features
3. A discussion of room/facility requirements
4. A discussion with the radiation physicist to verify operational performance requirements
5. A discussion with technologists to determine equipment capabilities and performance issues

After these topics have been discussed and fully understood, formal proposals must be requested from equipment manufacturers. This is accomplished by preparing a document that specifies equipment/department needs. This document will help the manufacturer understand more clearly exactly what features and options packages they need to price out for the buyer. Other purchase conditions should also be included. These may include such items as:

- Shipping charges to the room
- A 30-day evaluation period under normal clinical use, which begins after the equipment is satisfactorily installed
- Acceptance will be dependent on hospital's physicist's interpretation of equipment's functions measured against current or pending regulatory agency standards

This document is known as a *request for proposal (RFP),* and it is usually prepared by the department director. Some RFPs, particularly those prepared by government facilities, such as state-funded university hospitals, can be very complex and voluminous, covering more than 15 pages. At the other extreme, some RFPs are lacking in detail. In the author's experience, a three- to ten-page document, including financial spread sheets, should cover the necessary details for most any major equipment purchase. A sample of the essential elements of a well-developed RFP are shown in Figure 9-3. The RFP should be forwarded to at least three vendors. This increases the nature and scope of price negotiations, which works to the buyer's advantage. Generally, there is little advantage to involving more than five vendors because beyond this number, the process becomes very cumbersome, especially if a second qualifying RFP is issued. Vendors should be given a minimum of two weeks to forward their proposals to the hospital. The manner in which bid proposals are written and handled in many instances sets the tone for the balance of the negotiations.

Site Visits

Going on site visits to evaluate equipment can also be very helpful if they are coordinated properly. They are always time consuming and tiring, but they generally provide valuable reference information that can be used when final decisions are made. For a typical purchase, if five vendors are involved, three to five weeks will be needed to complete all the site visits. It is not unusual for such site visits to involve overnight stays.

It is generally advantageous to allow sales representatives to take the lead in arranging these trips. It is incumbent on them to find the most appropriate site to visit based on parameters set by the RFP. Two requirements may be that the sales representative arrange the visit to occur when procedures can be observed and that sufficient time be provided to the buyer to work with the equipment between or after these procedures have been completed. During a site visit, it is worthwhile for the buyer to have prepared as many questions as possible and to have an agenda typed or firmly in mind that defines the specific objectives for

Fundamental Elements to Be Addressed in an RFP

I. Conditions of Presenting RFP
- Date to be received by hospital
- Specify pricing to be for budget or bottom line price
- Number of copies to be provided
- To be delivered to whom at the hospital
- (Optional) Identify other companies who have been sent RFPs
- (Optional) Expected date hospital will make decision regarding vendor of choice
- (Optional) Principal or priority of points upon which decisions will be made

II. Description of Equipment
- Specify type or nature of procedures or tasks the equipment is to accomplish
- Identify who will be using the equipment (e.g., radiologists, neurosurgeons, cardiologists)
- Provide information if the unit will be used by personnel of more than one discipline
- Describe the environment where the equipment will be used (e.g., room size, degree of temperature and humidity control available, anticipated problems with eclectrical power supply)
- Specify operational features needed
- Specify important function parameters required while equpment is in use
- Considerations vendor will give to providing upgrades and equipment modifications
- Description of maturity of equipment with estimates of when significant changes in product design are expected or another generation of equipment is anticipated

III. Delivery and Installation
- Expectations regarding delivery and installation time frame
- Definition of lead time from after the order is placed
- Price includes FOB to site of installation
- Vendor's responsibility regarding assisting in the design of space preparation & cooperation with architect
- Penalties for not meeting agreed upon time tables

IV. Description of Term for Payment
- Definition of payment terms at (1) Payment with order, (2) Delivery, (3) Installation, (4) Final acceptance
- Definition of clinical acceptance period
- Description of who or which group of people has principal responsibility for accepting equipment and authorizing payment

▶ **FIGURE 9–3** Fundamental elements to be addressed in an RFP.

V. Conditions of Cancellation
- Descriptions under which the order in part or in total can be changed or cancelled and financial assessment on the buyer for making these changes

VI. Equipment Service
- Estimated cost of service contract; parts and labor separately defined
- Reasonable expectations regarding service response time with and without service contract
- Description of warrantee period and services provided within that period
- Equipment uptime guarantees
- Vendor's capability to provide both primary and backup service personnel on site
- Description of penalties to vendor for not meeting service obligations

VII. Inservice and Application Training
- Description of user training program to include number of visits from vendor's training personnel, paid trips that hospital personnel may take to other facilities to preview equipment's operational features while installation is continuing, and the total number of hours of onsite training that can be expected by the buyer

▶ **FIGURE 9-3** *Continued*

the trip so key questions and issues will not be forgotten. It is also worthwhile to have each vendor answer the same series of questions so that a thorough comparison of responses can be made at decision time. A written or mental agenda for a site visit may address the following elements, to be discussed with the equipment's users:

- Items not fully installed or known corrections not made
- Features most liked by user; most disliked
- Operational features that you feel are important

These are only the fundamental issues associated with the purchase of new capital equipment. Each department may have different criteria concerning new equipment, but the issues outlined here should be universally addressed. The author has seen many instances in which large sums of money have been committed to purchase equipment for the wrong reasons. As a result, the wrong features and even the wrong types of equipment were requested, which had a negative affect on the department's credibility and efficiency for several years. Sometimes, after seeing equipment in use, buyers may decide that consideration of alternate features may be important, and it is not unusual for buyers to modify their equipment specification lists and to send out revised RFPs. In this case, however, the list of manufacturers may be reduced to two primary bidders. There should be at least two bidders at this point, or all negotiating leverage is lost.

Negotiating the Purchase

After these site visits are made and the final proposals reviewed, it is helpful to prepare a grid that represents the key features and capabilities of each vendor's offering (Fig. 9-4).

Purchase Analysis Grid							
Characteristic	**Weight**	**Grade Vendor 1**	**Net Score**	**Grade Vendor 2**	**Net Score**	**Grade Vendor 3**	**Net Score**
Over Head Tube							
Heat Unit Capacity	5						
Rotor Speed	5						
Anode Composition	2						
Cooling Rate	2						
Sub Total							
Table							
Range of Tilt	3						
4 Way Float Top	2						
4 Way MotorTop	2						
Table Top Composition	2						
Smoothness of Tilt	4						
Sub Total							
Image Intensifier/TV Sys							
Maximum Image Size	5						
Alternate Sizes	4						
Overall Dimension of Image Tube	2						
Ease of Motion	4						
Signal to Noise Ratio	5						
Basic System Design	5						
Sub Total							
Spot Film Device							
Image Formatting	4						
Convenience	4						
Configuration of Radio Shield	3						
Sub Total							
Pacs Compatible							
Image Matrix	5						
Backup Disc Capability	5						
Number of Monitors	3						
Imaging Capability From Table	4						
Size of Monitors	4						
Sub Total							
Flouro Tube							
Heat Unit Capacity	5						
Rotor Speed	5						
Anode Composition	4						
Cooling Rate	2						
Table–Tube Distance	2						
Focal Spot Sizes	4						
Sub Total							
General							
Service Record of Similar Equip	5						
Stability of Manufacturer	5						
Perceived Support After Sale	5						
Sub Total							
Site Visit							
Ease of Installation	4						
Problems After Installation	5						
Service Experience	5						
Support From Manufacturer	5						
Were Customer's Expectations Met	5						
Sub Total							
Sub Total							

Weight x Grade = Net Score for Each Company

Weight = The relative importance of a given feature
Grade = Indicates the level each evaluator feels the equipment meets specification

▶ **FIGURE 9–4** Shows a grid that can be used to help sort out and define various features and capabilities of equipment that has been proposed for purchase by various manufacturers/vendors. Too frequently, what appear to be subtle or insignificant factors become embarrassing and politically expensive mistakes soon after first use.

This will help when comparing the features of each vendor's offering. The elements noted in this grid must reflect the key elements outlined in the RFP and vice versa; if they don't, more investigation or clarification is needed. Sometimes weighted values are applied to these elements to help quantify and evaluate the relative importance of various features. It is very important that each criterion and feature be fully represented in this process. It is not only important to evaluate equipment capabilities and features, but also it is important to evaluate each company offering a product. Each manufacturer has its own *personality,* which determines how it will deal with circumstances such as:

- Installation problems
- Flexibility in negotiating creative financing situations
- Timeliness of delivery
- Attentiveness to problems after the sale
- Flexibility in handling follow-up service problems
- Flexibility in writing low-cost service contracts

It is important for all involved to depersonalize the entire process of equipment evaluation and selection. It is the radiologist and the technologist who will be using the equipment routinely, and it is their daily needs, rather than the prejudices of the director and the physicist, that must be understood and given primary consideration. The director's and the physicist's roles in equipment selection are important, but not to the degree that they alone should determine what operational features and equipment capabilities are paramount. It is the author's opinion that the role of the director is to make sure that all the steps of the purchase process and considerations noted earlier have been accomplished and that the overall equipment acquisition process proceeds fairly, ethically, and in a businesslike manner. The director's final responsibility is to make sure that the actual purchase price and all related terms and conditions of the purchase are negotiated in a cordial but tough-minded manner.

A final decision should not be made without input from an experienced and capable service engineer. In many cases, these people know more about the idiosyncrasies of the equipment than physicists do. They are in contact with other service engineers, who may have experience with a particular piece of equipment or may have insights from their own experiences. This information can help the department to avoid the wrong purchase decision.

Sometimes substitutions or changes are necessary after the initial RFPs are received. Before the final purchase decision is made, each vendor must have an opportunity to understand the changes and to respond with a revised proposal, and the hospital administration has every right to expect the department director to maintain a level playing field for each vendor.

The role of a physicist in the equipment acquisition process varies considerably among hospitals. The radiation physicist should have an opportunity to review a draft of the RFP. In some instances, physicists will prepare the technical specifications that appear in the RFP. The physicist should have an opportunity to provide information about standards that must be met during postinstallation testing and final acceptance. It is most appropriate that the physicist indicate the technical performance parameters that will be used during his or her acceptance testing to minimize last-minute discrepancies in performance criteria that will affect equipment acceptability. These criteria must be included in the RFP before serious purchase negotiations occur (Fig. 9-5). Physicists can also provide important background information about the way the equipment is engineered and how these characteristics may affect image quality, dose, and reliability. Occasionally physicists want to specify specific internal components. Although this may have some merit in unique situations, standards regarding image quality, equipment flexibility, capabilities, and upgradability need to get pri-

Fundamental Elements of a Purchase Agreement

I. **Description of equipment:** Reference should be made directly to an edited and signed final copy of the vendor's proposal.

II. **Payment terms:** Amount of money to be included with order and a definition of all other increments of payment and the events that trigger such payments.

III. **Delivery:** Description of delivery date and date installation is expected to be completed, with clarification of penalties that would occur if these time frames are not met by vendor. Any charges that are acceptable to the hospital that are associated with delivery and installation should be defined.

IV. **Cancellation of order:** Clarification of terms and conditions under which the order may be cancelled with or without penalty.

V. **Service:** Clarification of term and conditions under which current and/or future service agreements are part of the purchase agreement.

▶ **FIGURE 9–5** Fundamental elements of a purchase agreement.

mary attention. As PACS Systems are integrated into radiology departments, connectivity with computer equipment is very important. Some departments have computer systems people who specialize in PACS technology. Because of the integration of PACS computer systems with X-ray equipment, their expertise is another important asset to developing equipment RFP and making the final purchase decision.

Installation and Final Acceptance Testing

A formal hospital acceptance procedure for all new equipment must be completed before that equipment is put into clinical use, but this should not occur until the machine is considered fully installed by the manufacturer. Once the hospital, through department recommendations, formally accepts the equipment, considerable leverage regarding any postacceptance adjustments is lost. The key is to understand what elements, features, or functions of the equipment may be subject to further refinement or improvement by the manufacturer. The manufacturer will be much more willing to take care of these adjustments to the department's satisfaction if they were appropriately addressed in the RFP. The acceptance process requires input from the following personnel:

- Radiation physicist
- Radiologist who will take principal responsibility for using the equipment
- Supervising technologist
- Service engineer (inhouse or under contract)

Unfortunately, the need for a formal acceptance process is often overlooked entirely or is incomplete, and this often leads to years of complaints from users and underutilization of expensive equipment. Indeed, the entire process of budgeting, determining needs, making the final selection, installing, and final acceptance must never be underestimated. Misguided purchases of even relatively inexpensive equipment can also lead to operational problems, utilization inefficiencies, and an unsatisfied staff.

We have not yet discussed price. Because negotiating price can be handled in several different ways, the subject will be discussed in very general terms. Closed bidding is one method of negotiation. This requires a carefully written and comprehensive RFP, which is submitted to each vendor. The RFP may be given to vendors during an open meeting at which the department's decision makers review and clarify each element of the RFP in an open forum with the vendors. The vendors have an opportunity to ask questions regarding any aspect of the RFP, including equipment features and installation and site planning issues. The vendors then prepare bid proposals based on what was said at the meeting and outlined in the RFP and forward them in sealed envelopes to the department. The department's representatives review these closed bids with the purchasing director and make their decision based solely on what has been written into the bid proposal. The closed-bidding procedure is most often followed by state and federal government-funded institutions such as veterans and military hospitals; state, county or city hospitals; and state university hospitals. Sometimes, the closed-bidding method is used to identify two primary vendors from the initial list of four or five vendors. This approach quickly limits the number of vendors without sacrificing the buyer's price negotiating leverage because the vendors all know when they receive the RFP that the first cut will be based both on the equipment's capabilities and features and on price. This leaves room to negotiate further refinements in price and equipment options. Negotiations from this point on will be limited to the two vendors whose bids reflected the most aggressive pricing and the most acceptable mix of equipment features and capabilities.

Most often, the closed-bidding procedure is not used. Generally, RFPs are mailed to vendors, who provide purchase proposals. The various proposals are reviewed by the department. Sometimes, the department's available funds are less than those initially anticipated for capital purchases. This situation creates a very different scenario that has too many alternatives to detail here. If a specific selection of equipment can be made, the vendor will agree to freeze the price for a future guaranteed delivery date until additional funds can be identified.

Needless to say, the variability of these situations can be great, especially in today's financial environment. There is one constant that should be kept in mind: vendors are as desperate to sell as buyers are to get as much as possible for their money. In such an environment, there is great mutual willingness to develop a wide range of creative purchase plans.

A final comment regarding the equipment purchase process: Given all the possible pitfalls, errors in judgment do occur. Such errors can result from a lack of skill or discipline during negotiations. Obvious departures from fairness by the vendor, the department, and, at times, by hospital administrators are not entirely uncommon. The amount of money involved in capital equipment purchases can be very large, especially when several systems are purchased at the same time. Also, the reputation and security of a salesperson within his or her company may be affected by the success or failure of a large sale. Hospital negotiators have a moral obligation to make a good deal for the hospital. They must keep open minds concerning particular vendors or machines until all questions have been asked and answers have been received. Consideration must go beyond the equipment. The stability and presence of the company must be evaluated as well. It is not uncommon to have a well-designed and well-built device leave the marketplace because the company went out of business or was purchased and dissolved by its new owner. These situations leave the hospital and department with an expensive machine that has no long-term support.

The rules of this game on the vendor's side are to be persistent and at times unrelenting in offering additional concessions, options, and discounting. The rules on the buyer's side is to consider all proposals in an up-front manner and to keep a level playing field during all negotiations. The terms of a deal can change at almost any time, but for the benefit of all involved, including the hospital, notification of these changes should be made available to all bidders and they should be allowed appropriate time to respond with revised purchase proposals. The final rule for the buyer is to keep all reasonable options on the table and under consideration until the final review of facts, features, capabilities, and final price is made. The final purchase decision should not be done in a vacuum. It is a given that the equipment being purchased will fail at one time or another and that it will not be universally liked by all users. For these reasons and for the sake of political harmony, the purchase decision should result from a consensus among key players. Finally, and perhaps most importantly, after the decision is made but before it is announced to the vendors, the director should complete a brief but detailed summary that clearly addresses the basic elements of the purchasing decision, including why the price is reasonable, answers to strong reservations regarding the final selection expressed by any of the key decision makers, and details of key points in the process that led to the purchase decision. Certainly all important criteria that had been spelled out in the RFP must also be satisfied.

PERSONNEL MANAGEMENT

Personnel issues have an immense impact on patient care, department efficiency, and the overall effectiveness of the services a department provides. It is as important to understand personnel matters as it is to understand the various historical, financial, and administrative aspects of operating a department. It is also important for all employees to understand that their value to the organization is in part affected by how they perceive and relate to the complex matrix of personnel issues surrounding them.

Any supervisor, manager, or director will readily agree that personnel management issues can pose the most challenging day-to-day problems. People may be considered to be the most valuable resource an organization has. This is true not only because of the services they provide, but also because of the impact they have on every aspect of the organization's daily operations as well as on the future success of the organization. Whether a specific management task involves developing new or changed policies, defining reporting lines, or—the three all-time favorites—establishing pay scales, implementing disciplinary action, and evaluating performance, the potential for loss of reasonable control and direction is ever present. People in management positions at all levels have therefore developed so many personal theories on how to maintain control that it is impossible even to consider a summary of these here. It is the author's view that success in handling these personnel management challenges is based on whether the manager is fundamentally secure with himself or herself and is sufficiently experienced to anticipate and deal with conflict. In addition, it is the author's opinion that the principal contributor to personnel conflict is rooted in a lack of perception and anticipation of problems. Certainly, good analytical and negotiating skills are also necessary once these problems materialize. The author has also noted that problems can result from a manager who is too confident about his or her philosophies and beliefs. Such confidence can prevent one from being open to new or different perspectives that could benefit the organization. It can also prevent one from developing a timely perception of impending personnel problems. Such confidence can also lead to a lack of sensitivity, which sometimes creates serious morale problems within an organization. The author has long recognized that there are very few pure right or best ways to approach or do something and that what is often more important is the attitude and quality of spirit that drives the manager. We have all witnessed managers who generate a sense of strength as a shield but who are actually driven by insecurity or may simply lack sensitivity or perhaps experience. Successful personnel management is built upon the following elements:

- Appropriateness of action
- Fairness and timeliness of action taken
- Courage to take action when necessary
- No surprises: keeping employees' informed of problems
- Genuine respect for employees' efforts on the job
- Enforcement of objectivity held by supervisors as well as by employees

Clearly, subjectivity, let alone prejudice, at any level when dealing with personnel issues is a convenience that neither the manager nor the organization can afford. One must always be asking what the underlying motives for taking any personnel action are and be honest and disciplined enough to listen to the answer and act accordingly.

Establishing Salary Rates

One of most obvious topics in personnel management involves establishing pay scales. The type of pay scale that is implemented will depend in part on how pay increases are handled. The management philosophy of the organization will determine how it views pay in relationship to performance. There are two basic approaches to this. One is to base pay raises strictly on performance, and the second is to base them primarily on longevity. There are also some methods that attempt to combine these two approaches.

Guideposts for Setting Rates

There always seems to be much speculation, if not suspicion, among employees about what criteria are used to establish their pay scales. In fact, only a few guideposts are used by institutions to help set pay rates for a given job. All these guideposts must be balanced by good judgment when deciding how they should be applied to any given situation.

We must assume at this point that job descriptions have been appropriately developed and that employees are familiar and comfortable with their job descriptions. It is important in some cases to write a job analysis, which is an important preamble to formulating a job description and contains a much more detailed, analytical definition of the job's characteristics. A job analysis also characterizes traits of employees who will be most successful in the job as well as the demands the job poses. Once this detailed overview is completed, a more concentrated summary of the job can be prepared, which is the job description we are familiar with. In many instances it is not necessary to write a job analysis.

Once the job description is finalized, the institution will generally refer to surveys prepared by consulting companies and by for-profit and nonprofit groups that provide salary information that are based on market surveys. They can provide objective comparisons of salary information that is received and reviewed by the human resources department with the radiology department director. Relatively recent legislation restricts the use of making phone calls to peers at other institutions on the basis that this represents price fixing. However, the federal government has instituted strict rules that outline how salary surveys may be conducted along with stiff individual and institutional penalties to be imposed if these rules are not strictly observed. Before making any attempt to gather salary information, managers should contact the human resources department for details on these rules. Most hospitals require the HR department to gather appropriate salary survey information.

The human resources director will meet with the department director to review and evaluate this information in light of at least three fundamental parameters:

1. Parity with similar positions that may exist elsewhere in the institution
2. Philosophy in terms of where the institution wants to be positioned in relation to other hospitals
3. Benefits offered in conjunction with actual dollars earned

Parity is achieved when pay rates are consistent among employees throughout an organization who have jobs with similar responsibilities. For example, ultrasound technologists who have the same level of certification should be paid the same whether they work in Radiology or in the vascular lab. Similarly, receptionists throughout the organization should be working at the same rate of pay if their individual job descriptions are similar. Parity is sometimes hard to judge because jobs may be similar but not identical. Accurate assessments, judgment, and fairness must drive the final determination of pay rates. Efforts to devaluate one group to save money almost always lead to unexpected expenses and chronic employee morale problems and sometimes even to legal action.

Each hospital determines whether it wants to pay high, average, or low salaries compared to other hospitals. This decision is purely at the discretion of hospital administration. One facility may view itself as a lean, hard-working organization and wants its employees to be compensated for working in such an environment by providing salaries at or above the 90th percentile. Another organization may believe that its employees benefited from the institution's prestige, high-tech profile, and provision of superior on-the-job experience and so did not need such high salaries. Still other facilities simply cannot afford high pay rates.

Benefit packages, which include holiday pay, sick pay, health care coverage, vacation pay, and other benefits, are offered in addition to base pay. From the employee's perspective, the benefit package should be considered as seriously as the base pay rate when comparing the facility's overall salary philosophy to that of other institutions.

Pay-for-Performance Model

As mentioned earlier, there are two fundamental philosophies regarding how a hospital will determine pay increases. The first is the pay-for-performance model, which is becoming increasingly popular. With pay-for-performance, a hospital uses clearly defined criteria for determining the amount of increase an employee is to receive. Sometimes this amount is derived by using a strict ranking format in which supervisors and the department director jointly determine the quality and quantity of each employee's work. Each job is given a single rate of pay, and increases beyond this "job rate" must be earned through performance. A cost of living adjustment may also be applied in addition to any raises based on performance. In some years, a 3% cost of living adjustment may be appropriate, while in other years no cost of living adjustment will be included. Thus an employee may have the following possibilities for pay increases:

- Job rate: As defined by the job description and the facility's philosophy on placement of salary scales
- Cost of living increase: Subject to the facility's financial strength and based on characteristics of the country's general economic condition
- Job performance: Based on an evaluation of the employee's overall quality and effectiveness of service

Under a strict pay-for-performance system, employees receive an annual performance review. All pay increases are based strictly on performance; however, performance must be

▶ TABLE 9−4
PAY FOR PERFORMANCE EMPLOYEE RANKING

RANK	% INCREASE
5	3.5
4	3
3	2
2	1.5
1	0

NAME	SECTION	RANK	NAME	SECTION	RANK
Namming W.	Rad Tech	5	Booker J.	Ulsd Tech	3
Anderson B.	Spec Tech	5	Leads H.	CT Tech	3
Allen R.	Transporter	5	Copland E.	Rad Tech	3
Brandy J.	Film Library	5	Shane I.	Film Library	3
Adler U.	CT Tech	4	Armor P.	NR Tech	3
Jamison T.	Reception	4	Paige C.	Film Library	2
O'Neal M.	Transporter	4	Timms R.	Rad Tech	2
Edgar G.	Reception	4	Spurn S.	N.M. Tech	2
Blair D.	N.M. Tech	4	Smith T.	Ulsd Tech	2
Twain H.	CT Tech	4	Johnson T.	Rad Tech	1
Trainer N.	MR Tech	3	Harrison E.	Spec Tech	1
Bonque S.	MR Tech	3	Adams W.	Film Library	1
Jones P.	Reception	3			

Employee ranking based on pay-for-performance criteria.

based on objective reasoning and discussions with employees throughout the year so employees are informed and are aware of their overall standing. Communication between the employee and the supervisor is crucial. These discussions are reviewed by the supervisor prior to completing the formal evaluation.

There are various methods that can be used to determine the specific amount of *merit* increase an employee will receive. One method used very successfully requires supervisors to group or rank all their employees into five levels, as shown in Table 9-4. In most instances and when large enough pools of employees are involved, prudent ranking will yield a distribution that resembles a bell-shaped curve. In other words, if the number of people assigned to each level is graphed, the graph would produce a bell-shaped curve with most employees placing in the level-three group. Each level is then associated with a predetermined percentage merit increase, as shown in Table 9-4. The percentage of increase assigned to each of the levels may change from year to year based on the organization's financial strength. For example, level three may yield an increase of 4% in one year, but in the following year may yield an increase of only 3%.

This ranking process forces an objective assessment of performance because the supervisor must evaluate each employee's performance in relationship to that of others in the department or section. Sometimes, the evaluation process requires both the supervisor and the employee to complete a performance evaluation form. The entries of both are discussed during the employee's performance meeting. In most instances, there is room for agreement and resolution of different grades. In other instances, more substantive disagreements occur which cannot be resolved. In this case, management authority gives the supervisor the option to determine the final grade. Based on individual performance evaluation meetings taking place over the course of the year, the supervisor will rank all employees when the personnel budget is prepared so that the appropriate increase will be available for each employee's anniversary date. In some institutions, all employees receive their performance increases at the same time of the year.

A number of elements should be reviewed when evaluating employee performance, including:

1. Personal traits: Includes such aspects as cooperation, flexibility, personal integrity, communications skills, and reliability

2. Technical performance: Includes the employee's understanding of theory and competence in applying theory appropriately to practical situations

3. General support given to the department mission: Includes the employee's understanding of the organization's goals and objectives and perception of how those goals can be successfully applied to patient care and to dealing with other customers

4. Interpersonal skills: Includes the employee's understanding of how his or her interpersonal skills affect patient care, the overall service provided to customers, and his or her success in dealing with coworkers

5. Areas of special consideration: Includes special efforts or accomplishments by the employee

Here too, subjectivity and prejudice at any level when dealing with personnel issues is not a convenience that the manager or the organization can afford. One must always ask what are the underlying motives for taking any personnel action. Anger based on any previous incident or on past performance does not serve the evaluator's or the employee's best interests. In fact, when disciplinary action is based on such anger, more serious personnel problems can almost be guaranteed. However, it should be made equally clear that not exercising legitimate authority when making objective and well-thought-out evaluations can create serious morale problems throughout the organization. To be sure, with authority always comes responsibility, and this is especially true when personnel issues are involved.

A crucial aspect of the pay-for-performance model is that all categories of employees have equal opportunity to receive the maximum merit increase because the amount of increase is based on performance of their individual jobs rather than on what the nature of those jobs are. For example, a clerical person, a technologist, and an escort may all be placed in the level-five group and receive the maximum percentage of increase that is associated with that level. The nature of the job has no relevance to the individual's performance. You must remember that the base job rate was established by the job description and not the amount of merit increase.

Another important element of pay for performance is that it helps develop a keen understanding that the value of individual performance is paramount.

Pay for performance also puts strength in the supervisor's evaluation and assessment of employees' performance and helps add a certain mindset within the organization in identifying performance as the prerequisite for increases. It also requires maturity and good judgment of management at all levels, and it can generate pressure on supervisors who must suddenly differentiate their employees' performance. This requires more analysis and careful placement of each employee in relation to the others. This method works best when department and section goals are clearly defined so that employees can anticipate and gauge for themselves the standard of performance that is expected by the supervisor.

► TABLE 9–5
INCREASES BASED PRIMARILY ON LONGEVITY

POSITION	1ST YEAR	2ND YEAR	3RD YEAR	4TH YEAR	5TH YEAR
Rad Tech	$14.25	$15.00	$15.80	$16.50	$17.15
NM Tech	$15.96	$16.80	$17.70	$18.48	$19.21
CT Tech	$15.53	$16.35	$17.22	$17.99	$18.69
Reception	$7.84	$8.25	$8.69	$9.08	$9.43
Film Library	$7.84	$8.25	$8.69	$9.08	$9.43
MR Tech	$15.53	$16.35	$17.22	$17.99	$18.69
Transporter	$21.38	$22.50	$23.70	$24.75	$25.73
Transcription	$9.98	$10.50	$11.06	$11.55	$12.01

An employee pay scale based on longevity.

Pay Increases Based on Time Worked

This second model usually assumes that each employee maintains a minimum performance level. There is not a single job rate per se. Instead, maximum and minimum pay rates are established for each job. Steps are established between these two points and are usually defined and spread at logical increments to produce a pay scale that is associated with years of service. The maximum pay rate is generally set at the fifth year, when the employee is "maxed out," as indicated in Table 9-5. Under this system, merit increases per se do not usually exist because, in practice, as long as a person continues to be employed, increases are likely. In fact, the criteria to receive an increase in pay are based on some combination of the employees number of years worked and ability to stay out of serious trouble. It is rare for an employee not to receive a pay increase that matches his or her longevity, whereas under the pay-for-performance model, a known percentage of employees will not receive performance increases.

The acknowledgment that an increase will be given to an employee generally occurs at the time of the employee's annual review. The performance evaluation is usually done using a standard form upon which characteristics, work habits, and other related elements are given numerical values. Supervisors are required to enter numbers that indicate specific performance characteristics. In some instances, the employee is given the same form to complete. In this case, the performance appraisal meeting between the employee and the supervisor is handled much as it is in the pay-for-performance model.

In both the pay-for-performance and longevity models, the evaluation can and should also be used to identify areas of performance that should be improved and to reinforce the potential for improving performance with specific objectives that are understood and mutually agreed upon. Unfortunately, far too many performance reviews are viewed by both supervisors and employees as rather nonproductive and ineffective encounters that are mandated by the organization rather than as opportunities to work out differences in perception between the supervisor and the employee. An effective meeting can help to establish better understanding between the two and, ultimately, a more pleasant and less stressful working environment.

Using Policies and Procedures as Effective Management Tools

It is difficult to evaluate employees' contributions to their jobs and to the mission and goals of the department unless both employees and their supervisors have a blueprint to fol-

Process for Developing New or Revised Policies

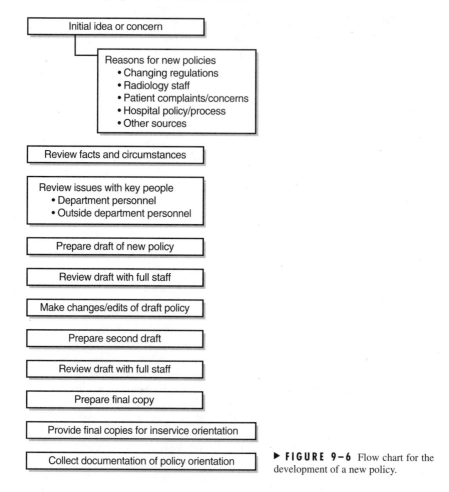

▶ **FIGURE 9−6** Flow chart for the development of a new policy.

low that provides some standards and expectations against which performance can be objectively gauged. Policies that are accurate, comprehensive, sufficiently detailed, readily available, and current must be in place. The department's operations committee or management group is the most appropriate forum for discussing and developing or revising department policies. Most departments have an array of policies and procedures. However, sometimes they do not reflect current practice. This creates opportunities for errors and a lowered level of performance and often, at least in part, accounts for the less than satisfactory performance of employees.

Copies of policies should be appropriately displayed throughout the department or otherwise available for quick reference. Sometimes, it is helpful to have a summary or abstract of each policy so that its essential elements can be reviewed quickly. Having policies immediately available in summary format encourages their use. Simple flow charts are also helpful and make interpretation easy. The flow chart shown in Figure 9-6 suggests an appropriate process for developing department policies. Figure 9-7 shows a policy for making policies.

Department of Radiology

Title: Defining Department Policies and Procedures

Policy: Any changes or affirmation of Department procedure that impacts operations or patient care shall be formulated using the procedure described below.

Scope: Includes all department employees, Department medical staff, and operational matters that may have an impact on the manner in which the Department is managed or patient care is provided.

Objectives: To provide a timely and consistent method for developing new or revised procedures within the stated scope of this policy. To develop an effective manner for distributing approved procedural information to all Department personnel and the Radiology medical staff. To establish a feedback mechanism to all Department members for acknowledging ownership and responsibility in observing the policy and stated procedures.

Procedure:
1. When a member of the management group or medical staff receives information that indicates a revised or new policy may be indicated, the information will be taken to the Department's Director or a Section Supervisor to present the matter for discussion at the weekly supervisor's meeting.
2. Based on available information, a draft policy with supporting procedures will be prepared by the Department Director. It is the responsibility of the Department Director or designee to assure that all appropriate Radiology and non-Radiology contacts have been made in an effort to gather background information that is needed to support the substance and appropriateness of the policy.
3. The first draft will be given to the management group and to the Department Chairman or designee for editing and discussion. These comments and further recommendations shall be returned to the Department Director within an agreed period of time.
4. The various comments and edits made on the first draft shall be discussed with the management group and Radiology medical staff. Comments solicited from non-Radiology personnel regarding the proposed policy shall be included to assure the impact of the new policy/procedures can be accurately estimated.
5. The comments and edits which have been forwarded to the Department Director on the first draft shall be incorporated into a second draft of the policy and again distributed for comment and edits as described above. This information is used to prepare a final draft for approval by the Director and Chairman of Radiology.
6. The approved policy is distributed to all members of the Department's medical staff, appropriate non-Department personnel, and Department Supervisors, who will discuss the policy in reasonable detail with their staffs. Each employee will acknowledge this orientation by signing a log sheet which is forwarded to the Department Director's office.

Date Approved   Department Chairman   Department Director

_____   _____   _____

▶ **FIGURE 9−7** A useful tool for establishing department policies.

Inservice Programs: Continuing Education

Inservice programs that offer a continual stream of worthwhile information to employees are an important aspect of personnel management. We will now discuss basic program requirements and highlight some of the advantages these programs offer. Any inservice or continuing education program should contain the following basic elements:

1. Variety of topics
2. Immediate application
3. Comprehensive and appropriately detailed information
4. Use of department, hospital, and outside resources to present programs
5. Inclusion of participation and follow-up to evaluate the impact of the program on operations in the department when possible
6. Question and answer session
7. Grading of each program

Continuing education programs should address information from more than one point of view. To help assure a balance of subject matter, topics can be grouped in the following ways (examples of topics are also given):

1. Immediate day-to-day duties
    - Safe use of oxygen regulators
    - Working with patients who are connected to respirators and monitoring devices
2. Purely technical
    - Improving image quality
    - New diagnostic procedures
3. General operational topics
    - Legal liabilities of employees
    - Policy review

These topics could be expanded and key people from other departments within the hospital invited to present discussions on personnel management, hospital finance, and general hospital administration. Over time, these presentations can provide employees with a greater awareness not only of their immediate work environment, but also of the bigger picture. Too often, the mistake is made that continuing education programs are not evenly distributed among technical and nontechnical personnel; it is also important that joint sessions are scheduled from time to time. Topics for programs for nontechnical personnel may include:

1. The mechanics of scheduling
    - Phone etiquette
    - How to handle difficult people on the phone
    - Contraindications of various medications
2. Escorting patients and body mechanics
    - Correct manner in which to move and lift patients
    - What patients want and don't want to know about the exams they are having in Radiology
    - How to answer touchy questions from patients about their doctors, their exams, and their diseases or conditions
    - How to answer questions about this hospital

3. Film library
- Statute of limitations and how it applies to medical records
- Legal implications of signing medical records out
- Legal implications of communicating diagnostic information to patients, physicians, or physicians' office personnel.

A continuing education program should also be developed for department supervisors and managers. Once again, there is a need to provide variety, application, and expansion of awareness in each of these sessions. Also, it is beneficial to invite other department directors as presenters to discuss mutual operational matters or to help iron out conflicts that may exist between the various departments.

Personnel Management: Taking Disciplinary Action

Sooner or later, circumstances will occur such that disciplinary action must be taken. Taking effective disciplinary action involves:

1. Open communication
2. Objectivity (nothing personal)
3. Respect for effort and work that is accomplished
4. Consistency of application
5. Courage
6. Timeliness and patience
7. A thorough review of current and previous incidents that affect the action being taken.

Open Communication

The best friendships can break down at times from a lack of good communication. The work environment seems to foster stress and create challenging situations among people who might not be friends, which increases the potential for miscommunication even more. It is no wonder that communication mishaps are so common in the business environment. Communication involves both sending and receiving messages. We tend to stress the former, but developing good listening and interpretation skills is at least as important. Sending complete messages is important because, if the sender fails to provide all the necessary information, the listener will have to fill in the gaps. The risks in doing this are clear.

On the other hand, the receiver must be patient and wait to hear the message in its entirety. Sometimes listeners will jump ahead and superimpose their views or what they are anticipating over what is actually being said. Listeners then end up with a combination of what was said and what they added or thought they heard.

The potential for communication errors goes well beyond these simple examples and the scope of this book. However, it is important to note that many, if not most, communication problems can be eliminated or reduced if we realize the potential for miscommunication always exists. This being the case, confirmation is needed. Positive closure on the conversation can be accomplished if the sender asks the listener to repeat or summarize what is being said, or by the listener saying or admitting he or she doesn't fully understand, and asking for clarification. These solutions are obvious. The problem is recognizing when this level of confirmation is needed at the time of the conversation, and then obtaining or giving the necessary clarification. It is here where perhaps the most effort should reside.

Objectivity

I can easily recall more than one situation when I found myself dealing not with the details of the situation, but with the person.

Harry is an individual with the capacity to broaden the definition of the rules a bit to conform to a particular situation. He called his work on a Monday morning after having been away the previous week at a family event out of town. The person at the front desk received the message that Harry had car trouble, and he could not get back to work as scheduled. Because of Harry's tendency to push the envelope on occasion, and because the floor was very busy that day, the on-duty staff was angry. The supervisor was urged to take care of this person and the supervisor, also aware of Harry's tendencies, brought the matter to the manager.

When Harry came in the following day, tanned from the sun, he was called to the manager's office for counseling. The manager expressed his views of Harry and how he operates. Then, without really listening, he gave Harry a chance to speak. After the explanation Harry received a written counseling report and promptly claimed that unfair management practices had been used.

The manager in this case was dealing with Harry and not the situation. If the situation was reviewed objectively and had been based on the specifics of the conversations and the facts a different result would have occurred. In fact, employees routinely called the front desk to say they are sick or that they have a personal emergency just as Harry did. Furthermore, Harry not speaking to the supervisor directly was a standard of practice of many employees in the department. If the specific events of the situation had been balanced with the standard of practice of other employees, the manager would have understood that Harry did not act improperly, since he did have car trouble.

Additional attention in this case should not have been directed at Harry, but at whether policy requires the message to be given directly to the supervisor, thereby avoiding the claim of unfair management.

A second example may help clarify the point. Mary requested and subsequently received a transfer from one area of the department to another. Although her work performance at the first location was problematic and generally unsatisfactory, no documentation existed to reflect this. After more than a year of satisfactory performance on the second job, Mary requested a transfer back to the first job when an opening became available. Many in the department knew of Mary's unsatisfactory performance in her former job and did not feel the transfer should be approved, but the policy was that internal transfers must be genuinely considered to qualified candidates before hiring from the outside.

Although it was tempting to yield to pressure from the employees and radiologists, looking at the situation objectively indicated that there was little basis to not allow Mary to transfer back to her first job, especially since no one else in the department had the necessary experience and training. It was necessary to deal with the situation objectively and not with employees' impression of Mary as an unsatisfactory employee. Although she was allowed to transfer back, Mary was subject to the hospital's three-month probation evaluation period. If Mary succeeded, the fear and assumptions would dissolve; if not, her employment would be terminated. It was important for Mary to understand the transfer carried some risk of long-term employment because of the three-month evaluation period, which should be put in writing.

Respect of Work Done

Having an appreciation for work done is, in part, an extension of maintaining objectivity. Despite a manager's feelings regarding an employee, the focus must be on the effort, skill, and quality of work that is accomplished. If employees and managers maintain this focus appropriately the potential for positive recognition is present and will serve the department and all concerned.

Consistency

Applying the same standard for performance is an essential lifeline for both employees and managers. Managers must be alert to dual standards and take appropriate action when necessary. Not doing so will eventually result in claims of unfair management practices and lead to significant problems regarding a lack of objectivity and perhaps prejudice. Maintaining consistency in policies and procedures is also essential for providing optimal service. All supervisors must make the manager aware of these potential double standards so that appropriate preventive action can be taken.

Courage

Courage is a key ingredient. Managers know the feeling when it seems all eyes and ears are anticipating what level of discipline will be taken. In both of the examples above, a group of people were, in a sense, eagerly awaiting the outcome. In other incidents the manager unilaterally sees the potential for problems and must take action. In the first example, the tendency is to overreact; in the second, the tendency is to wait and not to take firm initial action.

One can avoid overreacting by focusing on the facts and making sure communication skills are fully exercised. Maintaining a respect for work that was performed well also helps to put the current situation into proper perspective. To avoid problems that stem from not reacting soon enough, one must open lines of communication and be an especially good listener. Conversations with individual employees and in groups may be very helpful. Once the concerns are aired, an accurate interpretation is needed to assess the situation and to come to a fair conclusion.

Taking the lead and coming to a conclusion does require a measure of courage and fortitude. Because these decisions and conclusions cannot be "tried" each decision should be firm and able to withstand challenges.

Timeliness

Each profession seems to have a motto. In real estate, it's "Location, location, location." In personnel management, it may well be "Timing, timing, timing." I can recall almost as many times when exercising patience made all the difference as I can the times when taking prompt action was the most correct, if not the only, option. In the two examples above, not taking action early enough and conducting counseling sessions may have prevented the incidents from happening. On the other hand, overreading the significance of an event, acting on matters that are not important, or dealing with situations too soon is very discouraging to staff and only works to build resentment and distrust.

Perhaps this element of discipline depends on a manager's makeup more than in any other because it depends the most on individual judgment and interpretation of the circumstances. A healthy measure of self-confidence, and an awareness of basic principles, experience, and skill are essential ingredients for assessing timing. In short, one cannot make generalized guidelines as to when to take firm action or when to exercise patience, because every encounter or incident is different. It is, however, necessary that managers note that the concept of timing is as important as any other element to maintaining good morale and an effective level of services.

Keeping a Proper Review of Past Events and Good Communication

Finally, having an accurate understanding of a person's work history gives the manager a better perspective on the matter at hand. Without such a review the present discussion or counseling can get off track very quickly and yield unfortunate results. Knowing a person's work history requires proper documentation and the ability to access it quickly. Sometimes quick action is indicated and, if this information is not available, incorrect assumptions can result with negative consequences.

A conversation may need to be followed by subsequent rounds of communication that serves to enhance or qualify the message. The length of a communication is less important than the spirit or content it carries. A message can be overexplained or overstated. T. Haimann and R. Hilgert (*Supervision: Concepts and Practices of Management,* South Western Pub., Colorado, 1982) explain that poor communication can be adversely affected by:

1. Language interpretation
2. Status and position
3. Resistance to change
4. Indifference

Problems associated with *language interpretation* involve the use of jargon, terms that have multiple meanings, slang, and other figures of speech that can lead to different interpretations and incorrect conclusions. As a result, the intended message is sometimes lost. Communication between individuals who hold different positions within the organization can also cause problems. In this case, communication difficulties between, say, a boss and a subordinate may occur because each uses common terms in different contexts. Although clarification may be necessary, it may not occur because one of the communicating parties may fear appearing stupid if he or she acknowledges not understanding exactly what had been said. As a result, necessary questions are not asked and answers are not given.

Resistance to change is a very common communication barrier. If people do not want to participate in a particular situation, their passive and possibly negative feeling about what is going on will dampen the spirit of what is being said. In fact, sometimes the listener will cheat by deliberately taking what was said literally or reporting what was said out of context. Sometimes taking what is said literally without considering the spirit can distort the meaning of the communication and work to sabotage the message to the detriment of all involved.

Barriers to good communication also result from *indifference* on the part of the sender or receiver. Clearly, enthusiasm can generate significant positive chemistry between people who are engaging in a conversation. The presence of this chemistry can stimulate positive communication; however, its absence will often result in more mechanical or superficial discussion that usually results in only a part of the total message getting through. These missing pieces can lead to misunderstanding, confusion, and eventually a misinterpreted communication.

Clearly, the psychological makeup of the sender and of the receiver are an important aspect of good communication. In addition, the levels of their skill and awareness of techniques used to communicate are also important. It seems that some people are better at sending while others are better at receiving messages. This is also true when written communication is involved. An extended discussion of the psychological elements and the personal makeup of individuals in regard to communication matters is beyond the scope of this text. But you should understand that participants' security and level of esteem for self and others, as well as the value each participant attaches to the subject at hand, are essential determinants of how well a message can be sent and received. Carrying these concepts into our everyday activities in the radiology department can help to reduce errors and even to provide a more consistent service to patients. We have all heard the phrase "the chemistry is not good," and we have all seen the number of errors that can result when poor communication occurs. Given this, each of us must make a conscious effort to focus on the meaning as well as on the spirit of all communication. If we do so, the probability is that the essentials of what is being said will take priority over what is occurring at the personal level. It is the responsibility of each participant equally in communication to minimize the affect of these barriers on communication. Maintaining such a focus is not easy, yet it is essential.

What Is Personnel Management?

Hundreds of books have been written about management processes, techniques, and theories, and yet good management continues to be one of the most illusive elements of business practice. Millions of dollars are spent each year on seminars intended to train us how to develop and use successful personnel management techniques. Millions more are spent by employers to implement these programs in facilities throughout the world. Organizations are continually rediscovering that morale among their employees is less than optimal and continually move to revolutionize their entire practice in order to improve the current state of perceived morale. What is good management? Is it style? Is it simply exercising a logical approach? Is process more important than content or vice versa? One could continue with an additional page of questions regarding this topic. In the author's experience, any one of these or of a multitude of other questions will appear to be dominant at any one time in the course of an organization's maturation. It seems that by nature, people will continually reach for something that they perceive as better. In this regard, as one element of management practice is improved and accepted as standard, a new group of elements is identified. As an organization grows and matures, the needs of its employees evolve as well. Clearly, there are many needs in an organization, and, when examined specifically, the priority of these needs is in a constant state of change.

Balancing the Needs of the Organization and Those of Its Employees

Each organization has needs. Facility, space, and funding requirements must be met in order for it to support its mission. Sometimes, the needs of the organization and those of its employees may appear to be in conflict. In most cases, the problem may lie not so much in a specific condition as in a lack of sensitivity and wisdom concerning how to better understand this condition and to implement simple but effective solutions, and a lack of ability to mobilize employees to get involved in positive change.

Fundamental management techniques are equally essential to the overall success of a radiology service as are image quality, timeliness of diagnostic reports and the capability and scope of available equipment. Today, a new and significant element has been added to the mix of doing business in the health care industry: competition among a growing list of providers who are actively negotiating with HMOs and other payers for contracts that will help insure a future revenue stream to the hospital. This element has created tremendous financial uncertainty, pressure, and anxiety among all health care providers as they try. There is also a drive to produce more of a better service at a lower cost. It seems too often the case that "lower cost" is synonymous with "fewer staff." There is no hope of a provider meeting higher standards with fewer staff unless its managers and first-line employees practice good personnel management techniques, and unless retooled procedures and processes are as efficient and appropriate as possible. It is equally important for employees to recognize this effort by increasing their level of cooperation and the number of their suggestions to the extent possible.

Clearly, good management increasingly involves a process that involves team effort among the technical and nontechnical staff who must work directly with patients on a day-to-day basis. The concept of an integrated team effort must be a strong part of the entire management process. At no time in the past has the application of sound and effective management techniques been more important.

MANAGEMENT TECHNIQUES AND STYLE

Managers' specific roles will differ slightly between various institutions and even between sections within a single radiology department. As athletes vary in their abilities to perform in sporting events, managers vary in their abilities to provide strong and appropriate leadership. Haiman and Hilbert point out that good management does not necessarily come from "born managers," but rather from learned skills that are based on good, fundamental management principles. Delegating responsibilities and handling authority properly are critical management skills. In addition, the need for managers to develop a sense of objectivity and inner strength is essential.

Functions of Management and the Continuum of Management Activity

Management has been defined as getting things done through people. A *management cycle,* which identifies five distinct activities, has been outlined:

1. Planning
2. Organizing
3. Staffing
4. Directing
5. Controlling

We will proceed by discussing each of these activities in summary form.

Planning involves setting goals, objectives, policies, and budgets for an existing or new organization. It involves research and getting answers to many different questions. Planning is just as important when a new organization is being developed as when an existing organization is being reevaluated. A great variety of people should be involved to help brainstorm and to discuss ideas to the fullest extent. It also involves establishing goals and objectives.

Organizing defines which process will be used to accomplish objectives and goals. It also involves determining who and how many people will do the work, and it includes developing an organization chart that is used to establish lines of authority within an organization.

Staffing involves the acquisition and assigning of people to fill positions in all levels of the organization and establishes who in the organization has unique or special capabilities to accomplish each duty. Setting work schedules and evaluating appropriate staffing requirements are also important activities. It may also involve training personnel so they can meet performance criteria.

Directing relates to putting these resources in motion. Nothing important happens unless an organization has a sense of leadership. In some instances, direction must be obvious and strong, while in other cases, direction can be accomplished more quietly. It can be applied in a formal or an informal manner.

Controlling makes an activity meet prescribed standards related to a service's or product's overall quality, quantity, and timeliness. Controlling involves monitoring feedback, making decisions, and understanding when and how adjustments should be made. Controlling also includes continuously evaluating the appropriateness of current standards and defining new levels of performance when indicated.

Supervisors should understand the unique nature of each of these five management functions, and be ready to accomplish each one. Further, there is no beginning or end to the management process. These functions form a continuum of effort as supervisors and employees interact to keep operational goals on track. Over the life of an organization, greatest emphasis will be shifted from one to another of these functions. At one point, the organizational structure may need serious attention, while at another, controlling efforts may need to be strengthened. The director of this overall activity must be in a position and of a mindset to process as broad a spectrum of information as possible. In this way, the many aspects of the operation can be monitored and evaluated so that areas in need of improvement can be kept clearly in focus.

Authority Over and Supervision of Others

Having the authority to manage is having the power to give and enforce direction. Many people recognize two fundamental forms of authority, *formal* and *informal,* that occur in the workplace. Formal authority is the power that is passed to a supervisor by his or her superior, while informal authority is granted or voluntarily given by subordinates. Formal authority is demonstrated through organization charts, which delineate the chain of command. Such charts shows graphically who reports to whom and give some idea of the overall span of authority of each person noted. Having formal authority indicates that a person has a legal right and responsibility to provide direction and discipline; this right and responsibility are granted to that person by the organization. The organization must use this authority in accordance with federal and state legislation, for instance, right to work laws and wage and hour laws. These laws are reflected in the organization's personnel policies. Formal authority can also be delegated. A manager may delegate a portion of his or her authority to another individual. In this case, the second person has the power and legal support from the organization to direct the activities and actions of others.

Formal and informal authority can be equally effective and useful to the manager. There are many examples in which informal authority has had a much greater impact on a group of employees than has formal authority. The informal structure of an organization is as important to appreciate and understand as the formal structure, although it is often ignored. It can effectively challenge the formal structure of a given work group. Unfortunately, many managers view the informal structure as a natural enemy. But the astute managers can use the informal structure to advantage. The grapevine or rumor mill's effectiveness and efficiency in communicating information is sometimes unmatched. Unfortunately, the messages that are transmitted can be grossly inaccurate. There are many reasons why the informal structure is common to all organizations, and there are a number of reasons for people to join it. These include gaining

- Social contact
- Power

- Peer pressure
- Help in solving work problems
- Access to information ("being in the loop")
- Support

As noted earlier, some managers view the informal structure as a healthy and important part of an organization: it can generate significant pressure to make positive changes. Yet, its strength may also be a sign of ineffective management if it is not given the appropriate attention. In any organization, control of operations needs to be distributed in an orderly, logical manner, not as a result of the natural selection process of a pecking order.

If there were an informal organization chart, it would look very different from the formal organization chart. Here, power is distributed by pecking order among the participants, and sometimes the most significant leaders of the group can be the most unlikely. Like the formal structure, each informal structure has its own culture and personality. It is therefore not uncommon for an employee or group of employees to be victimized by the informal structure. In fact, employees sometimes leave an organization not because of dissatisfaction with the formal organization but because of the culture and spirit of the informal organization.

The Acceptance Theory of Authority

Exercising authority is sometimes associated with what is known as the acceptance theory. The concept here is that although legitimate authority can be exercised by a manager, from a practical perspective, authority must also be accepted by the employees. If this does not occur, authority will be severely diminished, often to the extent that there is little or no direction or leadership evident.

Delegating authority is an important process in management. Authority that is delegated should carry with it an equal measure of responsibility to provide leadership and direction and of freedom from significant second guessing and interference by the superior who has delegated the authority. Delegating authority without granting this level of freedom to direct and make decisions can be disastrous to both the organization and the manager involved.

Management Styles

Autocratic supervision is practiced by some managers in the belief that subordinates require strong and close supervision to achieve necessary productivity and quality performance standards. There is often a strong reliance and emphasis on rigid rules and discipline and decisions made without a reasonable degree of input from employees. This approach is sometimes seen as necessary to keep employees on the straight and narrow. The authoritarian approach is also referred to as classical management, which was an outgrowth of the industrialization the United States experienced in the early 1900s. Unions became strong, and it was widely believed that management and workers held inherently incompatible points of view regarding the work ethic. Management viewed workers as being interested in doing the least amount of work but getting the greatest compensation possible. Workers often saw management as having an interest only in productivity and maximizing profits at workers' expense. The basic theme was that one could gain only at the cost of the other. There was also a belief that job satisfaction and fulfillment are not necessarily important elements of the work experience. There was no attempt to seek subordinates' participation in decision making. In most work situations, employees find this approach to be frustrating and it can result in keeping employees at arm's length from the manager. General morale is usually low.

Other management styles adopt a more collaborative approach. Here, there is a general assumption that employees have a basic desire to do a good job and need direction and focus rather than discipline. Employees today are looking for ways to make their jobs more satisfying, and this need is more likely to be met by employing a style of management that focuses on employee needs in addition to organization needs. Unlike authoritative or autocratic managers, collaborative managers do not view management and workers as being inherently in conflict with each other. More and more managers are learning that the fundamental human needs of employees can be satisfied without giving up the store. In fact, there are many examples that clearly show when these needs are satisfied, the overall performance of employees and the organization as a whole increases substantially. Employee cooperation and flexibility also increase. Clearly, accomplishing any appreciable level of synergy between management and employees requires a measure of maturity in both groups. It also involves a well-thought-out plan that has been developed through the active participation of both groups. Such a plan can take the form of an operations plan or of some adaptation of such a plan.

Each manager eventually adopts a style that fits his or her personality and maturity level and is not in conflict with his or her level of self-confidence. The theory X and theory Y managers were first described by Douglas McGregor. These models are at each end of a spectrum that spans the distance between total authority at one end and collaborative management at the other. Theory X managers exhibit a strong autocratic approach that depends on discipline, and theory Y managers depend more on collaboration and on clearing road blocks so that their employees can perform required duties. There are relatively few managers who are purists and hold entirely to either the X or the Y model; there is rather, usually a blend of the two in each manager but a tendency toward either the X or the Y approach.

Interestingly, many managers are not fully aware of their own orientations. Many theory X managers, for example, tend to view themselves as theory Y managers. One way to understand a manager's orientation is to use a managerial grid. The managerial grid was developed by Robert Blake and Lane Mouton to describe various levels and styles of management (Fig. 9-8). Five significant managerial characteristics are positioned on the grid and the manager plots his/her personal beliefs accordingly. If a manager objectively places him or her self on this grid, they can better understand their own particular style. Although this may be a little risky, and potentially embarrassing, a manager might ask his/her employees to plot the prevailing management style on a similar grid.

Motivation and Maslow's Hierarchy of Human Needs

One of the best-known concepts in management is Maslow's hierarchy of human needs. Dr. A. H. Maslow was a well-known psychiatrist who studied elements that contribute to motivational energy in people and found that this energy related to basic human needs. He developed a progression of human needs, which is shown in Figure 9-9. Maslow concluded that there are five fundamental levels of needs that exist in people and believed that human nature is such that we are all driven to satisfy those needs. Further, he believed that if these needs are not satisfactorily met, significant dissatisfaction results and our interest in accomplishing tasks diminishes—in other words, we are not motivated. These needs range from the most basic human needs, which he called physiological, to the highest, which he described as the need for fulfillment.

MANAGERIAL GRID

Country Club Management

Thoughtful attention to needs of people for satisfying relationships leads to a comfortable, friendly organization atmosphere and work tempo

Team Management

Work accomplishment is from committed people; interdependence through a "commonstake" in organization purposes leads to relationships of trust and respect

Organization Man Management

Adequate organization performance is possible through balancing the necessity to get out with maintaining morale of people at a satisfactory level.

Impoverished Management

Exertion of minimum effort to get required work done is appropriate to sustain organization membership

Authority–Obedience

Efficiency in operations results from arranging conditions of work in such a way that human elements interfere to a minimum degree

---

▶ **FIGURE 9–8** A managerial grid that indicates several approaches that evolve over time and become management styles.

Maslow connected the human requirement to satisfy these needs to motivation and adapted this philosophy to the work environment. His conclusion was that the human requirement to satisfy each of these levels of need creates motivation. Once a level of need in this hierarchy is met to a satisfactory degree, people seek the next level until they eventually reach a sense of fulfillment. Motivational energy draws us to find or create ways that will lead us to the next level of satisfaction. Once we have satisfied our physiological and safety needs, we are driven to look toward the next level. Maslow's theory helps us to understand how managers can view motivation in their employees.

Maslow's progression of human needs also suggests that each person will establish different personal criteria for satisfying each level. For example, one person's needs for security might be satisfied by $5,000 in a savings account and a full-time job at a local family-owned hardware store, while another person's needs for security might not be met until he or she has $100,000 invested in secure stocks and a job in a Fortune 500 company. This diversity of criteria indicates the complexity of human nature and also points out that there is no one formula that can be applied to satisfying all employees' needs.

Yet, the hierarchy of needs can be applied in the workplace. One of the traps managers can fall into is to assume that they are solely responsible for motivating employees. According to Maslow, motivation to a large degree comes from within. Each person, whether on the job or in private life, calibrates his or her individual needs with the five fundamental human requirements described by Maslow. In other words, every person may have a need to satisfy each of the five levels, but each person will define or perceive differently what he or she will specifically require to satisfy his or her needs. Managers and employees should consider three aspects of this. Two have already been noted: first, there is no single formu-

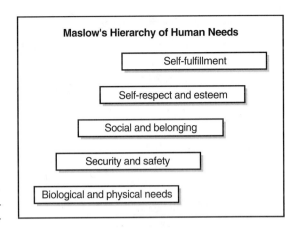

FIGURE 9-9 Shows Maslow's hierarchy of human needs.

la that will determine how a given individual will view a satisfier of need, and second, each of us has a hierarchy of needs that must be satisfied in some way. Given that motivation occurs primarily from within, the manager's job is to create an environment at the workplace that offers as many reasonable opportunities for each employee to tap into as possible. If this effort is recognized by employees, they will generally appreciate the manager's efforts and should be expected to respond positively. If this effort is not sensed by employees, either the manager's effort was misguided or the employees need to understand better the realities of what is possible in that particular work environment.

There are many other motivational theorists. M. Drafke describes several others in "Working in Health Care." Behaviorists such as E. Mayo, M. P. Follett, D. McGregor, C. Argyris, and F. Herzberg all have slightly different positions but all recognize specific motivators that people naturally respond to. Another group of famous theorists, H. Fayol, M. Weber, F. Taylor, and H. Gantt, viewed motivation as derived, or at least strengthened by, management structure rather than by the human needs.

You will recall an earlier statement that good managers are not born but made. A manager must learn to recognize and blend these and other motivators to create a positive work environment. The object is to encourage employees to exercise their positive motivational energy through an enriched work environment. Employees have equal responsibility to realize that they must work with these opportunities in the most positive manner. It is sometimes beneficial to keep in mind that human nature is not perfect, and there is no reason for either managers or employees to anticipate perfection. The objective is to develop a spirit in the workplace that encourages cooperation and positive motivational energy. Right and wrong are less important than creating a positive spirit and confidence in mutual effort.

Both employees and managers must create and direct workplace activities and systems so that people can attain a basic level of fulfillment on the job without losing control of the operation. We all recognize that this is not a terribly easy task. It requires employees to participate in the development and implementation of policies and programs that in aggregate will improve the culture of the organization and patient care.

Another approach to understanding human motivation is shown in Figure 9-10. Here we see that Maslow's five-level hierarchy has been compressed into two levels. In addition, this model suggests that human needs do not necessarily occur in a predetermined progression. The second level consists of three basic needs (social, esteem, and self-fulfillment). The theory behind this model is that a person will often average his or her varying

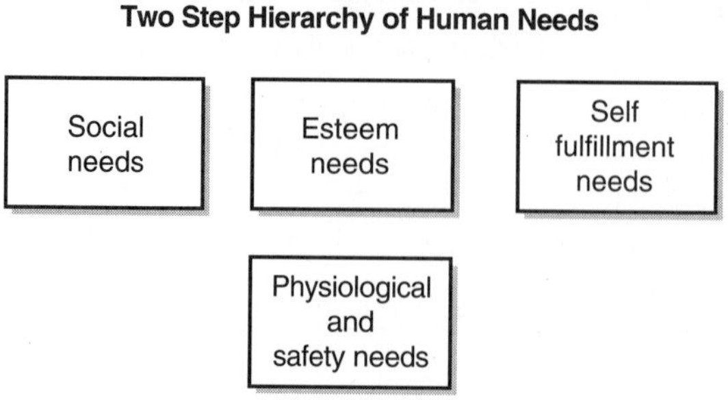

Two Step Hierarchy of Human Needs

| Social needs | Esteem needs | Self fulfillment needs |

| Physiological and safety needs |

▶ **FIGURE 9-10** Shows a variation on Maslow's hierarchy of human needs.

degrees of fulfillment in each of these elements to create a combined effect that is generally viewed as a feeling of overall satisfaction or dissatisfaction. We must keep in mind that each person will define their own satisfiers of need.

Conclusion

This brief discussion about motivation is meant to demonstrate that there are many nonmedical aspects of work that require at least a basic level of understanding and appreciation. Both managers and staff are encouraged to seek out and read more about motivation. In a radiology department, there are many opportunities for supervisors, managers, and employees to make opportunities that can improve overall services, improve job satisfaction, and enhance patient care. Fortunately, a career in radiology provides an extremely wide variety of venues where one may find a satisfactory level of fulfillment, and it is well worthwhile to fully test as many of these areas as possible. This not only benefits the employee, but also strengthens the institution. Indeed, radiology management involves far more than the mechanics of budgeting, radiation safety, and equipment acquisition and the dynamics of moving large numbers of people through complicated procedures each day. Each manager and employee has the responsibility to take full advantage of every opportunity to work together to reduce unnecessary stress and improve the overall service.

STUDY QUESTIONS

1. Briefly describe the following elements of an operating budget:
   Line item
   Overhead
   Accrued expenses
   Direct expenses
   Indirect expenses

2. Briefly describe the importance of performing each of the seven steps discussed in the chapter while developing an operating budget.

3. What are variable and fixed expenses? Give an example of each and explain how the two examples have to be calculated when developing a budget.

4. Why are final capital budget approvals by the hospital based on the mission statement of the institution?

5. Briefly explain each of the seven criteria for approving replacement equipment purchases.

6. What questions should be considered when requesting a replacement piece of equipment versus an additional machine?

7. Briefly explain one or two problems that can result if department budget requests are too conservative. Give examples.

8. Five steps were defined as necessary preliminary groundwork for preparing to acquire capital equipment. Briefly explain why each of these five steps are important to complete.

9. Which of the two major methods would you use to establish pay scales for your employees? Briefly explain the reasons for your choice.

10. What are some of the pitfalls commonly encountered when writing personnel performance appraisals, and how can they be avoided?

11. Give some examples of pay scale issues that relate to the issue of parity.

12. Briefly explain why each of the seven basic elements defined in this chapter is important to an inservice program.

13. Provide four topics for inservice/continuing education programs for the two groups shown below. Use topics other than those described in the text.
    Reception
    File clerks

14. Briefly explain why each of the seven steps regarding effective disciplinary action are important to observe. Select one and explain what can happen if it is omitted.

15. Give a brief explanation of why communication breakdown between individuals occurs.

16. What do we mean by management style?

17. Briefly describe and explain each of the five functions of management.

18. What is the difference between informal and formal authority? How do they rank in importance?

19. Do you believe that Maslow's hierarchy of needs actually applies to everyday management situations?

Radiology Services Provided by Freestanding Facilities

O B J E C T I V E S F O R S T U D Y

After reading this chapter, the student will

▶ Appreciate why freestanding radiology facilities have become so common.

▶ Appreciate some of the advantages and disadvantages that these facilities offer patients.

▶ Understand some of the advantages and disadvantages to working in freestanding facilities as compared to working in hospital-based departments.

▶ Appreciate the marketing efforts that must be made by these facilities to assure continued referrals.

▶ Understand the need to balance patient volume with payer mix and collection rates.

▶ Understand the basic requirements involved in developing floor plans for these facilities.

▶ Understand some of the basic arrangements hospitals and groups can establish in order to develop and operate such a facility.

INTRODUCTION

Although we usually think of radiology work being performed in hospital-based departments, many radiology procedures are performed in private office settings. In fact, many radiologists who practice in freestanding offices have no hospital affiliation whatsoever. Other radiology groups have contractual agreements with hospitals that permit them to operate radiology services both in a hospital and in a freestanding private office. In some instances, as we will see later, hospitals have "joint ventured" with radiology groups to form separate corporations that then establish and operate freestanding facilities. Freestanding radiology facilities may be located several miles from the nearest hospital or on a hospital campus.

WHY THESE FACILITIES HAVE BECOME SO POPULAR

The number of freestanding outpatient radiology offices began to grow rapidly in the early 1980s. There were two important reasons for this. The first is that operating a private office affords a group a level of autonomy that it does not experience with a hospital-based practice. Decisions concerning buying new equipment, establishing pay rates for employees, determining the number of employees, and when to make renovations, for instance, are all driven solely by the group because there is no managerial affiliation with or accountability to a hospital. In addition, operational philosophies and decisions regarding medical practice and protocol can be quickly implemented because there is no need for hospital review and approval. Moreover, many groups have moved to operating outpatient facilities in order to protect current and future revenue. A hospital facility, for example, may not be capable of handling additional volume, so new referrals may be sent elsewhere. This affects not only the hospital's revenue, but also the practice.

FREESTANDING FACILITIES AND THE PROSPECTIVE PAYMENT SYSTEM

As the impact of DRGs began to be felt in the early 1980s, the threat of decreased hospital inpatient revenues caused anxiety among hospital administrators. They began to see the need to increase their own outpatient activity to help offset anticipated losses resulting from declining inpatient volume. Today, as a result of the prospective payment system, hospital-based radiology practices must rely on the hospital to make contractual agreements with HMOs; they may not believe that their own interests are appropriately represented. Every financial agreement that the hospital signs for its in- and outpatient services binds the practice as well whether the agreement is advantageous or not. As hospitals reacted to the new prospective payment laws in the early 1980s, radiology groups became less confident that their financial interests would be optimally served. As a result, contract negotiations between radiology practices and hospitals began to take on a more urgent and focused tone. Some radiologists eventually won more flexibility and were able to establish practices in private offices while continuing their commitment to provide in patient services at the hospital. This environment provided the practice with a degree of financial independence and some security, which fostered an entrepreneurial spirit. This spirit eventually resulted in some radiology groups leasing or purchasing space immediately across the street from their own hospitals in order to capture outpatient business.

Some hospitals signed contracts that allowed radiologists to open outpatient facilities only beyond a given distance to reduce the chance that hospital patients would be drawn there. Other contracts had provisions that required right of first refusal: Before the practice can open a private office, it must first offer the hospital a partnership interest. If the hospital declines, the group may proceed.

THE CORPORATE STRUCTURE OF PRIVATE PRACTICES

Once it has been determined that a proposed office meets the requirements of the contract with the hospital, planning may proceed to find funding to build the facility and buy equipment. This can be accomplished in a variety of ways. If the facility is to be wholly owned by the practice, funding commonly comes from a bank loan, accrued savings, combining with a group of outside investors (venture capitalists), or some combination of these. A venture capital group is a group of people who pool their money for the purpose of investing in new business ventures with the intent to gain returns through profit from each business's operations and/or to reduce their overall federal tax liability.

Because such medical groups function as private corporations, they must operate the financial aspects of their services under the same federal and states laws as any private for-profit corporation. The corporation is required to pay taxes and is subject to all personnel wage and hour laws. Patient care must meet prevailing standards of care criteria.

Group practices generally have blanket insurance contracts which cover liability for the radiologists and their employees. It is worthwhile for employees to verify insurance coverage at the time of employment, however. The law is clear that patients may bring legal action against any member of the staff. In fact, some technologists have purchased insurance to protect themselves from significant losses resulting from unfavorable judgments. Ironically, the fact that an employee is protected by his or her own malpractice insurance sometimes increases the probability of being named individually as a defendant. The same holds true for employees working in hospital-based departments.

There are two fundamental types of litigation that patients may pursue. One is criminal and the other is tort action. Criminal litigation occurs when a patient charges that wrongful acts have been committed that violate state or federal laws, while tort litigation involves personal injury or losses. Tort situations include injury or personal losses resulting from:

- Misconduct (intentional or unintentional)
- Negligence (intentional or unintentional)
- Breach of duty
- Not using reasonable or prudent judgment
- Departure from standard of care

Tort law provides for compensation to correct or mitigate the personal loss, while criminal law primarily provides for punishment through incarceration and sometimes through compensation in addition to incarceration. Criminal acts are violations of state or federal statutes. Murder, larceny, and theft are examples of criminal acts. These are referred to as acts against the state rather than against an individual. *State* in this case may refer to either federal or state bodies. In most instances malpractice complaints are litigated torts unless unusual circumstances can be identified or claimed that involve deliberate acts as opposed to issues such as poor judgment or a lack of skill or competence.

REFERRALS AND A NEW EMPHASIS ON SERVICE: GETTING AND MAINTAINING BUSINESS

Every business must provide services and/or goods in order to generate income. Naturally, this income must be greater than expenses to assure the continued operation and growth of a company. In the case of an outpatient facility that provides radiology services, business comes in the form of patients who are referred by physicians outside the radiology group. Thus, referrals are the lifeblood of an office practice. Competition among private offices to gain these referrals is high. Offices usually try to position themselves based on the following elements:

- The scope or variety of services that they provide
- The perceived level of care given the patient
- The proficiency and friendliness of the staff
- The quality of diagnostic consultation provided
- The number and type of complaints from patients back to referring physicians about the level of care patients believed was provided

In addition to these five elements, there is a business chemistry that seems to connect referring physicians to the people in radiology offices. In an outpatient setting, the strength of the radiology service depends heavily on this chemistry. It is important to realize that this chemistry is dependent not only on the radiologists and on the quality of the group's interpretations, but also on the technical, clerical, and management staff. Usually, if patients complain that they have been treated in an inappropriate manner, referrals will eventually decline.

It is crucial to remember that patients cannot easily evaluate the quality of medical care they receive. They don't understand radiographic quality, equipment, and film, but they are very aware of the manner in which they have been treated by the staff and the general conveniences that they have been offered. The appearance of the office and how comfortable they feel in the office are also very important matters that help patients determine whether they liked the experience and whether they will complain to the doctor who referred them to the office.

WHAT SERVICE IS ACTUALLY PROVIDED

Over recent years, the concept of product lines in health care has emerged. It is true that the product may not take shape as a specific item on a shelf or in all instances be tangible. Nevertheless, services rendered can be considered products. This emerging point of view of product-of-service reinforces the sense that medicine is driven at least in part by strong business elements.

Many people in health care feel that the service they provide is more personal and should not be referred to as a product. This seems especially true when the patient needs special personal attention because of the nature of the procedure or service being performed. It is, perhaps, not as important to acknowledge a product line per se as it is to identify and analyze the service provided. It is important for each person who provides medical services to understand the importance of his or her individual role in working with the patient as an individual who requires a professional approach mixed with the human touch.

It is difficult to establish when sufficient chemistry between referring physicians and a provider exists that it actually generates new patient referrals (business). It is, however, easy to find reasons why referring physicians should not send patients to a particular facility. It is clearly the responsibility of each staff member, whether in a hospital or an office setting, to contribute his or her best efforts toward working with patients in the most positive manner possible and to the highest level of quality attainable.

REIMBURSEMENT FOR SERVICES PROVIDED

Billing for outpatient services is a complex function because of the many different payer plans that are available to patients. The importance of payer mix and collection rates to hospitals was discussed in Chapter Five. These factors apply equally to outpatient facilities. It is important for everyone who works in private office practices to be aware of who specifically is paying for each service because these payers are customers in close partnership with patients and referring physicians. All payers either have or are developing quality control programs, and all of these programs include methods for screening patient complaints about the services their contracted physician groups provide. When a current contract with an HMO runs out, the probability that the HMO will be willing to renew the agreement will in part depend on these factors.

CONFLICTS REGARDING SELF-REFERRALS TO PRIVATE OFFICES

The movement toward capturing a growing outpatient business in private offices gained considerable momentum beginning in the mid 1980s. Freestanding diagnostic radiology facilities seemed to pop up everywhere. The number of facilities that were founded by nonradiology physicians also increase rapidly between 1980 and 1990. As a result of this, some referral patterns changed. Nonradiology physicians and group practices who had large enough patient bases entered into partnership ventures with radiologists to build private offices that provided radiography and other services. This created what is referred to as self-referred patient activity: Physicians could see patients in their offices and then send them to radiology facilities that they partially owned.

The proliferation of freestanding outpatient facilities increased further with the addition of MRI and CT installations during the mid 1970s and 1980s. This proliferation was in part because many hospitals had to apply for approval through the certificate of need (CON) process, which could delay the start of construction by a year or more. Physicians were able to take advantage of their "CON-free" status because they operated in freestanding outpatient settings: Outpatient facilities are not subject to CON laws, and, therefore, physicians were able to move quickly and could install CT and MRI scanners without delays. The high cost of acquiring such equipment encouraged many partnerships between radiology groups and hospitals. Under this circumstances, hospitals could provide the lion's share or all of the cash needed to build, equip, and open the office. Both parties benefited because the hospital billed for their technical fees and the physicians billed for their professional fees, just as in hospital-based services.

SAFE HARBOR LEGISLATION

The vast majority of these facilities were operated by ethical physicians. However, there was growing concern about referrals to facilities that were co-owned by nonradiology practices or individual nonradiology physicians. To a degree, the revenue received by these investors was dependent on referral patterns that they themselves could generate or control. The number of inappropriate self-referrals may have been relatively small; however, such abuses did occur. Facilities that had competent and highly skilled radiologists generally attracted sufficient business on the basis of quality of service. These practices are busy enough and don't need to supplement their regular referral base by recommending inappropriate studies. As more of these facilities formed, third-party payers, including the federal government, became concerned that unnecessary tests were being ordered by physicians who benefited from the revenue they generated for the private radiology facility.

These concerns resulted in a federal law—known as safe harbor legislation—that was signed by President Bush in 1992. It prohibited partnerships between facilities and individual physicians and physician groups who would send patients to those facilities for testing or treatment. More dramatically, there was no grandfathering provision, which meant that any functioning radiology facility that had the potential for self-referral must be restructured so the referring groups could not benefit financially from sending patients to that facility.

ADVANTAGES OF FREESTANDING RADIOLOGY FACILITIES

Outpatient radiology diagnostic centers can provide a substantial benefit to patients. First, these facilities are generally in more accessible locations and have available parking; some even offer escort/transportation services. They are also usually much smaller than the average hospital-based outpatient facility, so patients who cannot walk easily are able to reach the facility with less difficulty. In many instances, outpatient radiology offices are in the same building as the patient's physician, which provides additional convenience. Also, in these instances, X-ray film, reports, and medications can often be picked up or delivered by the patient with a minimum of difficulty, delays, or walking.

THE NATURE OF THE WORKPLACE

Most employees who work in private offices feel that the office environment is more intimate than hospital-based radiology departments. This, of course, can be considered an advantage by some and a disadvantage by others. There seems to be little difference in the amount of work performed by technologists in hospital-based departments and technologists in private radiology facilities. However, those who feel more comfortable in an office environment often cite a more casual and predictable work environment. Also, compared to those in hospital-based departments, a technologist in a private facility might share in nontechnical chores such as reception, transcription, and film-filing work. Questions concerning basic activities such as ordering supplies and equipment can be discussed more directly with physicians or the office manager, who have direct authority to purchase items and are unfettered by the cumbersome processes that are present in hospitals.

Hospital-based departments provide a broad spectrum of services. Intramural competition and territorial issues become very important in hospital-based departments, and they are almost always more complex functionally and politically than are private offices. Policies and procedures sometimes seem to abound in hospital-based departments because of the broad range of customers and of services provided. The degree of dependence on others to perform their jobs well in other sections of the department increases in hospital-based departments, and this dependence can create a degree of pressure and intensity that may not exist in a private office setting. The more people working in the department, the less autonomy one has. Some people work better with increased autonomy, while others do not, and hospital-based departments generally offer less autonomy to employees. Furthermore, one finds a large cadre of hospital physicians, including residents and medical students, which can increase frustration levels.

Despite these pressures, the overall activity generated by hospitals does create a certain excitement that attracts technologists to hospital-based programs. In addition, technologists feel the challenge that is associated with handling inpatients and the emergency/trauma cases that are common in hospital-based departments. There is also greater opportunity to increase personal and professional growth through additional training. Hospitals usually install new technology and implement new diagnostic and treatment procedures before private offices do.

There is no clear consensus among technologists regarding whether working in offices or working in hospital-based departments is more desirable. As we have seen, each has its characteristic advantages and disadvantages, which should be considered carefully before one accepts an offer of employment. Pay rates are generally comparable, although benefits sometimes differ considerably.

MARKETING PRIVATE OFFICE SERVICES

It is critical not only to maintain present patient volume, but also to increase income to cover growing personnel expenses, equipment costs, and routine office operating expenses such as rent and utilities. Referral patterns develop over long periods of time and are the lifeblood of an outpatient facility. The present level of competition for private outpatient referrals makes it imperative that each employee accept a new obligation toward working with patients in a proficient, professional, and friendly manner.

As HMO and PPO plans cover more and more patients, marketing efforts by private offices have substantially increased. These marketing efforts should highlight efficient patient scheduling, short patient wait times, fast report turnarounds, and convenient hours. Such competition occurs not only among private offices. Hospitals are similarly increasing their efforts to maintain present patient referrals and are trying to attract back as many outpatients as possible from private offices by signing aggressive contracts with HMOs, PPOs, and other payers. Hospitals have learned to leverage their ability to offer many other services at the same site. Lab, radiology, physical therapy, and other services are all available in the hospital, and many hospitals are renovating these areas to be more outpatient-friendly. It is to the HMOs' and PPOs' benefits to contract with facilities that offer the widest range of services to their subscribers. Private offices have a limited scope of services. What they do provide must be the best possible.

OFFICE FLOOR PLANS

Floor plans for private offices will vary significantly depending on the range of equipment used and the number of examinations performed. Several freestanding radiology facilities are as large as some hospital-based radiology departments. The floor plans shown in Figure 10-1 is from a moderately large facility.

Some of the most important considerations that should be taken into account when developing an outpatient facility are sometimes overlooked during the design phase. Such considerations include the number, location, and size of patient and staff toilet areas. Appropriate space for separate, gowned female and male waiting rooms is also an important consideration, along with the number, size, location, and type of patient lockers and changing areas. A facility should also carefully separate as much as possible staff activities from patient routes between reception, changing, gowned waiting areas, and X-ray exposure or scanning rooms. Staff work areas need to be arranged and located in such a way as to prevent patients from overhearing conversations among staff. It is very important that appropriate storage areas be programmed into the architectural plan. The film file area always

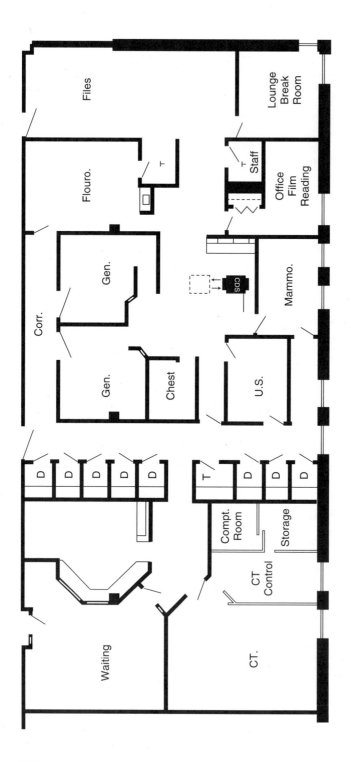

OUT PATIENT CENTER

▲ **FIGURE 10–1** Shows the floor plan of a successful outpatient radiology facility that offers a wide range of services. This floor plan can support approximately 15,000 exams per year. As freestanding facilities grow to this size and larger, the overall level of activity often requires a more defined division of responsibilities between technical and clerical personnel. (Courtesy of Medical Imaging of the Lehigh Valley.)

seems to be overcrowded in these facilities, and certainly an appropriately sized and pleasant room should be provided for staff lunch and break times, which can also double as a meeting room. A private area for managers' offices, where business and personal conversations can be conducted with appropriate privacy, is also important.

HOSPITAL-OWNED OUTPATIENT FACILITIES

Hospitals, too, have built outstanding freestanding facilities, primarily to define and protect their current service area or to claim new referral territory. Many of these facilities include lab services as well as radiology, respiratory procedures, physical medicine, and pharmacy departments. Some hospitals have built their diagnostic centers at long distances from their primary locations. Such a satellite facility can serve as a mini-network to patients who live close by. Once a patient receives services from one of these satellite facilities, the probability that he or she will seek service at the parent hospital increases. Having a number of these satellite facilities scattered throughout a large area potentially increases negotiating power with HMOs because of the patient access such a network provides.

These satellite facilities often have space available for physician offices. If the base hospital has a good reputation and if it can encourage members of its medical staff to see patients in these facilities, another referral stream can be established, which leads to new inpatient volume. Such a network may also attract other providers who are looking for cost-effective and convenient locations at which their patients can receive medical care.

These arrangements can be especially advantageous to physicians who are looking to expand their practices because hospitals will often charge physicians a lower-than-average rate to rent space. The hospital benefits because there is a significant possibility that the physicians' offices will generate referrals. There is also value in the good will these arrangements can produce throughout the community.

S T U D Y   Q U E S T I O N S

---

1. List three reasons that radiology groups develop and operate freestanding facilities.
2. List four factors that can be used to evaluate the quality of service provided in a freestanding facility. Explain what strategy you would use while negotiating a contract with an HMO to provide radiology services for its subscribers.
3. Why was safe harbor legislation implemented?
4. From a patient's perspective, what are the advantages and disadvantages to using services in a freestanding facility?
5. How would you market your services to referring physicians you have already established good relationships with and to physician groups that do not currently refer patients to your facility?
6. How does payer mix affect the profitability of your facility?
7. Give one fundamental difference between corporations and partnerships.
8. Describe some key issues that need to be considered when setting up a freestanding outpatient practice.

INDEX

Note: Page numbers in *italics* refer to illustrations; page numbers followed by t refer to tables.